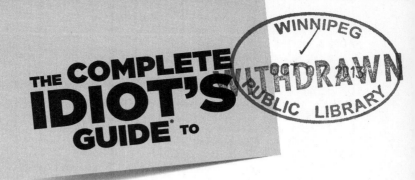

THE COMPLETE IDIOT'S GUIDE® TO

The pH Balance Diet

by Maria Blanco, CFH

ALPHA

A member of Penguin Group (USA) Inc.

ALPHA BOOKS

Published by Penguin Group (USA) Inc.

Penguin Group (USA) Inc., 375 Hudson Street, New York, New York 10014, USA • Penguin Group (Canada), 90 Eglinton Avenue East, Suite 700, Toronto, Ontario M4P 2Y3, Canada (a division of Pearson Penguin Canada Inc.) • Penguin Books Ltd., 80 Strand, London WC2R 0RL, England • Penguin Ireland, 25 St. Stephen's Green, Dublin 2, Ireland (a division of Penguin Books Ltd.) • Penguin Group (Australia), 250 Camberwell Road, Camberwell, Victoria 3124, Australia (a division of Pearson Australia Group Pty. Ltd.) • Penguin Books India Pvt. Ltd., 11 Community Centre, Panchsheel Park, New Delhi-110 017, India • Penguin Group (NZ), 67 Apollo Drive, Rosedale, North Shore, Auckland 1311, New Zealand (a division of Pearson New Zealand Ltd.) • Penguin Books (South Africa) (Pty.) Ltd., 24 Sturdee Avenue, Rosebank, Johannesburg 2196, South Africa • Penguin Books Ltd., Registered Offices: 80 Strand, London WC2R 0RL, England

International Standard Book Number: 978-1-61564-305-9
Library of Congress Catalog Card Number: 2013933134

15   14   13   8   7   6   5   4   3   2   1

Interpretation of the printing code: The rightmost number of the first series of numbers is the year of the book's printing; the rightmost number of the second series of numbers is the number of the book's printing. For example, a printing code of 13-1 shows that the first printing occurred in 2013.

Printed in the United States of America

Note: This publication contains the opinions and ideas of its author. It is intended to provide helpful and informative material on the subject matter covered. It is sold with the understanding that the author and publisher are not engaged in rendering professional services in the book. If the reader requires personal assistance or advice, a competent professional should be consulted.

The author and publisher specifically disclaim any responsibility for any liability, loss, or risk, personal or otherwise, which is incurred as a consequence, directly or indirectly, of the use and application of any of the contents of this book.

Most Alpha books are available at special quantity discounts for bulk purchases for sales promotions, premiums, fund-raising, or educational use. Special books, or book excerpts, can also be created to fit specific needs. For details, write: Special Markets, Alpha Books, 375 Hudson Street, New York, NY 10014.

Publisher: *Mike Sanders*
Executive Managing Editor: *Billy Fields*
Senior Acquisitions Editor: *Brook Farling*
Production Editor: *Jana M. Stefanciosa*
Cover Designer: *William Thomas*

Book Designers: *William Thomas, Rebecca Batchelor*
Indexer: *Tonya Heard*
Layout: *Ayanna Lacey*
Proofreader: *Krista Hansing*

Contents

Introduction

If improving your health in the most natural way possible is important to you, you've come to the right place. In this book, I share all the health benefits of balancing your pH through diet and simple self-care—you'll find the results phenomenal and far reaching. In this book, you discover how easy it is to alkalize your life, learn how to check and maintain that wonderful balance, and 101 exciting recipes to help make it all happen.

The pH balance diet focuses on consuming simple, natural foods humans have eaten and thrived on since time began. It teaches you how to eat healthily and abundantly for a lifetime, while you naturally avoid many illnesses and chronic diseases.

In the recipes in this book, you discover the basis of real nutrition. You'll finally lose those nagging cravings. You'll achieve a level of wellness you might have never thought possible. And if you're overweight, you'll be astonished at how fast your weight goes down, even as your energy levels soar.

How This Book Is Organized

I've divided this book into three parts to make it easier for you to find the information you need to learn how and why the pH balance diet works and to tailor a plan that's right for you. Each part provides foundational information, hints, and tips on which to build:

Part 1, What the pH Balance Diet Is All About, explores the scientific concepts of pH, including relative acidity and alkalinity, and how these relate to your health. You learn why the standard American diet (SAD) contributes to imbalances that lead to disease, and how balancing your pH via the foods you eat can prevent and correct those imbalances.

In **Part 2, Making the pH Balance Diet Work for You,** you discover the many foods, supplements, and activities that put your health goals within easy reach, and I give you a step-by-step plan to put your body's pH to work for you. You also learn how to check your own pH and adjust your diet to achieve your goals. I also provide an abundance of food-prep tips to help you succeed on the pH balance diet.

Part 3, pH Balance Recipes, is where I share 101 pH balance recipes for juices, smoothies, and desserts, and I offer menus for a crowd as well as for one. From grab-and-go to sit-down meals, Part 3 has you covered.

At the back of the book, I've included resources for further reading, hard-to-find nutrition supplements, pH testing equipment, unusual foods, and lots more.

Extras

Throughout the book, I've included extra info in sidebars. Here's what to look for:

ACID ALERT!

Heed the warnings in these sidebars that can affect your health or seriously compromise expected results.

BALANCE BONUS

Check these sidebars for hints that make balancing your pH easier or advice that increases your understanding of some subject.

DEFINITION

These sidebars provide the meaning of terms relevant to the topic at hand.

PHABULOUS PHACT

Look here for interesting and helpful information on pH, nutrition, research, and expert opinions.

Acknowledgments

This book is dedicated to all people who suffer from diseases and disorders rooted in malnutrition, whether acquired through toxicity, insufficiency, or overconsumption. —*Ad Majorem Dei Gloriam, Anno Domini MMXIII*

Very special thanks go to Marilyn Allen of Allen O'Shea Literary Agency and to Brook Farling, my acquisitions editor at Alpha Books, for having such faith and confidence in me and for their warm support and expert guidance throughout this project.

To my friend, Dr. James Pendleton: many heartfelt thanks for reviewing this book for accuracy and offering the benefit of your insights as both writer and physician.

Finally and foremost, a deep, heartfelt *thank you* to my husband, Dewayne, and to our children, who have unwaveringly supported me through my writing endeavors and who have been tireless cheerleaders for "the cause" that they may not have always understood. And to my son, Joseph: many thanks for your generous transcription assistance when my eyes refused to uncross!

Special Thanks to the Technical Reviewer

The Complete Idiot's Guide to the pH Balance Diet was reviewed by an expert who double-checked the accuracy of what you'll learn here, to help us ensure this book gives you everything you need to know to adopt and thrive on a pH balance diet. Special thanks are extended to Dr. James Pendleton.

Dr. Pendleton is a primary care physician specializing in a naturopathic approach to family medicine. He has nurtured a family practice in Seattle, Washington; directed a VIP medical center in Abu Dhabi, United Arab Emirates; and designed innovative nutritional supplements for manufacturers and markets throughout the world. He is an assistant professor and has taught college sciences at several institutions, including Bastyr University, where he received his training in primary care naturopathic medicine. He earned his bachelor of science in microbiology from Florida Atlantic University and served as a military paramedic.

Trademarks

All terms mentioned in this book that are known to be or are suspected of being trademarks or service marks have been appropriately capitalized. Alpha Books and Penguin Group (USA) Inc. cannot attest to the accuracy of this information. Use of a term in this book should not be regarded as affecting the validity of any trademark or service mark.

What the pH Balance Diet Is All About

In Part 1, we explore the role pH plays in maintaining health and how the concept of the pH balance diet came about. I share some basic science explaining what pH is and how it can affect your body's ability to maintain a healthy balance.

Then we look at why the standard American diet is not healthful according to the pH balance theory and how that theory came about. You also learn how to determine whether your body is suffering from hyperacidity, as well as various methods of cleansing and alkalizing your system.

Finally, you learn to prepare yourself for adopting the pH balance diet.

Balance in Life and Aging

In This Chapter

- A primer on pH
- The properties of acids and bases
- Your body's slight alkalinity
- Reaching a healthy pH

Nearly every week, a new diet is introduced and hyped, and inevitably, people try these diets, often with little success. Unfortunately, what most all these diets have in common is that they lack a single vital element—balance. Low-carb diets, for example, are often too heavily weighted toward proteins and fats. Low-fat diets often contain excessive amounts of starches and sugars. The list goes on and on. Striking the right balance is important for success in dieting—and, in fact, in every facet of your life.

Balance is everywhere in your life. When you breathe, you take in oxygen and exhale carbon dioxide and other waste products. Without completing both actions, neither is helpful or beneficial for very long. You spend your days maintaining a balance of wakefulness and sleep, work and play. Your body's systems have regular cycles of taking in nutrients, assimilating them for building and repair, and eliminating the resulting waste. Remove any one of these processes, and the entire system becomes imbalanced, breaks down, and ceases to function.

So it goes with diet. Balance exists in all things, and the balance of the body's pH is no exception.

What Is pH?

In chemistry, *pH* (or potential of hydrogen) is a relative measure of how *acidic* or *alkaline* a substance is on a scale of 0 to 14, with 0 being the more acidic end of the scale, 14 being more alkaline, and 7 being neutral, or neither acidic nor alkaline. To get technical, the pH scale is logarithmic, so a pH value of 4 is 10 times more acidic than a pH of 5, a pH of 5 is 10 times more acidic than a pH of 6, and so on. The pH of pure water is normally 7.

DEFINITION

pH is a notation for the *potential of hydrogen* and refers to the concentration of hydrogen in a solution. An **acid** is a chemical substance that has a value of less than 7 on the pH scale. Acids are proton donors that can neutralize alkaline solutions (bases). An **alkali** is a chemical substance with a value greater than 7 on the pH scale. Alkalis, or bases, are proton acceptors and can neutralize acidic solutions.

When discussing pH in relation to your diet, we're looking at how food and beverages impact the acidity or alkalinity of your body, its tissues, and its tissue fluids.

When you consume a certain food or drink, your body has a specific reaction to it. Every food or drink produces an acid-forming or alkaline-forming action as a result of that food's mineral residues. Lemon juice, for example, is an acidic liquid, but the mineral residues resulting from consuming lemon juice are alkaline. Therefore, lemon is an alkaline-forming food. Meats, dairy products, many nuts, seeds, and legumes decompose to leave an acidic residue, so eating too much of these can disturb your body's pH balance and shift it toward the acid end of the spectrum.

Irish writer and hobby-chemist Robert Boyle first referred to substances as either acids or alkalis (bases) during the seventeenth century, when he noted that certain substances tasted sour, corroded metals, and turned litmus paper red. He similarly noted that the alkalis felt slippery, turned litmus paper blue, and lost some of these properties when combined with acids.

Nearly 200 years later, Swedish scientist Svante Arrhenius hypothesized that water could dissolve chemical compounds into individual ions and that acids caused the release of hydrogen ions into solution.

In the late nineteenth century, Danish chemist Soren Peder Lauritz Sorensen studied the effect of ion concentration on proteins. While doing so, he discovered that the relative concentration of hydrogen ions was important, and to give meaning to the measurement, he created the pH scale to serve as a simple representation of hydrogen ion concentration.

To this day, the pH scale is still one of the most basic tools of chemistry and is indispensable in medicine and other sciences— including nutrition.

A Look at Acids

With opposing properties, acids and bases have the ability to neutralize one another. Perhaps you'll recall from elementary science classes that adding baking soda (sodium bicarbonate, a base) to vinegar (an acidic solution) produces a spectacular reaction. When the baking soda encounters the vinegar, it receives H+ ions from the solution and rapidly releases carbon dioxide, bubbling and quickly overflowing its container.

When combined, the sodium bicarbonate (baking soda) and acetic acid (vinegar) produce sodium acetate and carbonic acid. The carbonic acid then decomposes into water and carbon dioxide, and it's this process that neutralizes the acid in the solution and causes all the foaming.

The Properties of Acids

As Sorensen discovered, acids can be either weak or strong, and their concentration can be diluted by the addition of water. Stomach acid, which works together with certain enzymes such as pepsin to digest proteins, is an extremely strong acid with a pH value that normally ranges between 1 and 3.5. This high level of acidity is necessary for breaking down the food you eat into their component amino acids so your body can use them.

> **PHABULOUS PHACT**
>
> Stomach acid causes proteins in your food to twist out of their normal shape. This allows the enzyme pepsin to break them down into smaller, usable peptides.

By the same token, if you drank a half-gallon of water as you ate a steak dinner, your stomach would have difficulty producing enough acid to overcome that volume of water and break down the steak. In fact, if you've ever experienced the discomfort of indigestion after a protein-heavy meal and an evening of drinking, you may have unwittingly caused it by consuming too much fluid too near the time of your meal.

Whether they're weak, strong, or somewhere in between, all acids share similar characteristics that make them easy to recognize:

- They have a sour taste.
- When applied to a wound, acids produce a sharp or stinging pain.
- Acidic solutions turn litmus paper red.
- When they react with metals, acids produce hydrogen gas.
- When they react with carbonate bases, acids produce carbon dioxide gas.

Common Acids

Lemon juice and vinegar are two common acids that are easily recognizable by their tastes. The following table shares some other common acids.

Common Acids

Acid	Chemical Formula	Found In
Acetic acid	$HC_2H_3O_2$	Vinegars, marinades, salad dressings, condiments
Carbonic acid	H_2CO_3	Carbonated water, soft drinks, blood buffering agents
Citric acid	$H_3C_6H_8O_6$	Citrus and other fruit juices, added flavorings
Hydrochloric acid	HCl	Toilet bowl and masonry cleansers; naturally occurs in the stomach's digestive juices
Lactic acid	$HC_3H_5O_3$	Naturally fermented pickle products, yogurt, and similar foods; also a pain-producing waste product found in muscle tissue as a result of overuse
Nitric acid	HNO_3	Chemical fertilizers, wart removers
Phosphoric acid	H_3PO_4	Soft drinks, jellies, preserves, pet foods, some cleaning agents
Salicylic acid	$C_7H_6O_3$	Aspirin; corn and wart removers; medications for fever, pain, and inflammation
Sulfuric acid	H_2SO_4	Batteries, air pollution, acid rain

A Look at Bases

While acids are formed by H+ ions in solution, bases are formed when chemical compounds break apart to form a negatively charged hydroxide ion (OH–) in water. The strength of a base is determined by the concentration of hydroxide ions in the solution. The more concentrated OH– ions, the stronger the base.

Because they neutralize one another, bases, or alkaline substances, can be thought of as the opposite of acids. But that doesn't necessarily mean they're preferable to, or safer than, acids. Both strong acids and caustic bases can be corrosive in nature, and depending on their strength, they can do considerable damage. The key to whether they're dangerous lies in how highly concentrated they are and in their ability to be balanced or reasonably neutralized.

The Properties of Bases

Let's look at one common base—household bleach. Just a drop of the undiluted chlorine bleach you use in your laundry can strip the color from and eat a hole right through a brand-new pair of jeans in a matter of minutes. Chlorine bleach is such a strong base, it can dissolve your skin and hair cells, too. Yet a proper dilution of chlorine can be added to drinking water to kill various *pathogens* that would otherwise pose a serious threat to your health.

DEFINITION

A **pathogen** is usually a microscopic organism (a germ) such as a virus or bacterium that can cause disease. Fungi and yeast can also become pathogenic.

Like acid substances, alkaline substances share a common set of attributes:

- Bases have a bitter taste.
- Bases have a slippery feel to them. Think soap.
- Bases turn litmus paper blue.

Common Bases

Lye, soap, and chlorine bleach are three common alkaline substances found in the home. The following table describes several others.

Common Bases

Base	Chemical Formula	Found In
Ammonia	NH_3	Gaseous ammonia is sometimes used as an inhalant to revive people who have fainted; liquid (anhydrous) ammonia is used in chemical fertilizers and grease-cutting agents
Ammonium hydroxide	NH_4OH	Glass and window cleansers, other cleaning solutions
Calcium hydroxide	$Ca(OH)_2$	Skin astringents that tone and contract pores
Magnesium hydroxide	$Mg(OH)_2$	Some antacids and laxatives, such as Milk of Magnesia
Potassium hydroxide	KOH	Soap- and textile-making applications
Sodium carbonate	Na_2CO_3	Detergents; commonly called soda ash
Sodium hydroxide	$NaOH$	Lye, soaps, oven cleaners, drain cleaners
Sodium phosphate	Na_3PO_4	Degreasers, detergents

Your Body's Narrow pH Margins

pH isn't relevant only in the fields of chemical engineering and industrial applications. Everything—even the tissues within your body—has a pH value. And as you can gather from some of the examples discussed in the previous section, the wrong pH value in the wrong place can do considerable harm.

You'd never consider drinking a caustic drain cleaner because, if you did, the cleanser would dissolve all the delicate tissues in your esophagus and you'd likely die. By the same token, your stomach lining is perfectly suited to the highly acidic environment of the hydrochloric acid it produces to digest your food, but a similar concentration of acid in your bloodstream would certainly kill you.

All your bodily tissues and organs must operate within a very tightly controlled pH range, and that range differs according to the tissue, the work an organ performs, and the body's various needs.

The normal pH ranges for human tissues and secretions are listed in the following table.

Normal pH Ranges

Tissue	Normal pH Ranges
Bile	7.00 to 7.70
Blood, arterial	7.40 to 7.45
Blood, capillary	7.35 to 7.45
Blood, venous	7.30 to 7.35
Brain	7.10
Feces	4.60 to 8.40
Gastric (stomach) juices	1.00 to 3.50
Heart muscle	7.00 to 7.40
Liver	7.20
Pancreatic juices	8.00 to 8.30
Saliva	6.00 to 7.40
Skeletal muscle	6.90 to 7.20
Small intestine	7.50 to 8.00
Urine	6.80

PHABULOUS PHACT

A difference of 1 on the pH scale is a pretty big jump: a pH value of 1 is 10 times more acidic than a value of 2, 100 times more acidic than a value of 3, 1 million times more acidic than a value of 7, and 10 trillion times more acidic than a value of 14!

As you can see, most of the body's tissues are normally slightly alkaline. The major exception is the gastric secretions of the stomach and, to some extent, the other organs and secretions associated with digestion. (More on this in the next section.) Suffice it to say, when the body's tissues and secretions don't fall within their normal pH ranges, the processes they're responsible for are performed less efficiently, or not at all.

Internal Hygiene

To maintain general health and proper tissue and organ function, your body carefully regulates your blood's acid/alkali balance. Your lungs, skin, and kidneys all work together through a variety of equilibrium, or balancing, processes to keep everything in check.

In fact, your body can go to extremes to try to maintain pH balance. *Ketoacidosis* (diabetic acidosis) is one of the most dangerous possibilities for a diabetic and usually occurs when blood sugar levels have risen too high and go unregulated for too long due to a lack of sufficient insulin.

DEFINITION

Ketoacidosis, or diabetic acidosis, is a dangerous condition that may occur in people with diabetes when the body cannot use sugar (glucose) as a fuel source because there's little or no insulin available and fat is used for fuel instead.

Insulin normally works to regulate blood sugar levels, but it also regulates the storage and burning of body fat. When insulin levels drop to dangerously low levels, the body begins burning huge quantities of fat for energy, even though blood sugar levels are high and continue to rise. At this point, an overaccumulation of acid-forming sugar begins spilling out of the blood and into the urine, thanks to the kidneys, along with excessive newly formed ketone bodies that also have an acidifying affect in the body.

Then the lungs are employed. The body tries to reduce the level of acidity by increasing respiration—even to the point of panting. With each exhaled breath, the body expels acid-forming carbon dioxide, and the increased respiration helps reduce blood acidity for a while.

Meanwhile, the kidneys are still filtering at maximum capacity, dumping high volumes of glucose (sugar) into the urine. This causes large amounts of water and alkaline salts to be lost through increased urination. This is now a real crisis that will cause dehydration. Dehydration causes further concentration of acids in the blood. Eventually, breathing and urination become inadequate to control the acidosis, blood acidity exceeds its normal bounds, and without emergency medical intervention, death could be the result.

Now, granted, that's an *extreme* example of how the body attempts to put out-of-whack pH levels back where they belong, but the body continually works at less intense levels to maintain this delicate balance. While ketoacidosis is a rapidly advancing acute crisis, chronic low-grade acidosis is an ongoing process that, over time, can deteriorate health and shorten lifespan. If you continually bombard yourself with acid-forming foods and drinks, high stress levels, and inadequate or extreme levels of physical activity, over time, you'll create an internal environment that makes maintaining your acid/ alkaline balance difficult. If not corrected, eventually your health will suffer.

To avoid this, your body is perpetually at work maintaining pH at acceptable levels in all your various tissues, primarily through processes of elimination, the utilization of buffers, and diet.

The Importance of Your Elimination Organs

Two primary causes are at the root of nearly all diseases:

- Deficiency, or the lack of essential nutrients
- Toxicity, or the buildup of poisons in the body's tissues

Your body has three primary avenues to eliminate toxins—which includes overly acidic substances:

- Your kidneys
- Your lungs
- Your skin

The kidneys help detoxify the blood by removing excessive solid (fixed) acids through the process of urination. The lungs work to balance the body's pH through normal respiration. They're able to eliminate gaseous (volatile) acids that form during normal metabolism when carbon dioxide mixes with water in the blood to form carbonic acid. To a lesser degree, the body is also able to sweat out a certain amount of toxic acids through the skin.

PHABULOUS PHACT

Carbon dioxide (CO_2) is the product of efficient cellular respiration. When fuel (fat or glucose) is burned in a cell, CO_2 diffuses out of the cell into the red blood cells (RBC). There, an enzyme called carbonic anhydrase converts it to bicarbonate (a major buffer for pH), which is then released back into the blood and floats freely until reaching the lungs. In the lung, the bicarbonate goes back into a RBC and is converted into CO_2. When you exhale, this CO_2 diffuses out and across the cell membranes and out of the lung. Very little CO_2 is dissolved in the blood.

Together, your kidneys, your lungs, and your skin work to reduce toxins and maintain your body's pH balance.

Your Body's Mineral Stores

Given the proper balance of nutrients, including alkalizing minerals, the body is able to maintain a healthy state beginning at the cellular level. Under balanced conditions, cells are able to take in nutrients and rid themselves of waste easily and efficiently. But when the body becomes overburdened with too much acidic waste, or when cell membranes are "locked" and can't let in nutrients because they're clogged by stubborn fluid retention, that's where problems begin.

Your body must maintain the proper pH balance in all its tissues in order to survive, so it'll do everything in its power to correct the problem. It starts by drawing on its mineral reserves to neutralize acidity in the blood and other tissues. Calcium is one of the most abundant minerals in the body and is found mostly within bones. It also happens to be an important alkalizing mineral. So excessive acidity in the blood can be balanced by calcium drawn from your bones.

In fact, if you eat a diet too heavy in acid-producing meats and other proteins, carbonated drinks, sugars, chemical additives, and preservatives, your body will draw on its calcium and other mineral reserves to create a buffer against the effects of that high acidity in the blood. This calcium enters the bloodstream and is dissolved in your tissue fluids to neutralize excessive acidity, but what happens to your bones?

Over time, your mineral reserves are depleted by your body's desperate attempts to maintain balance. Osteoporosis, diabetes, certain cardiovascular diseases, cancers, and kidney disease are but a few of the debilitating diseases that occur and progress when pH is chronically out of balance and cannot be corrected because either the organs that regulate pH are exhausted or the body's reserves of mineral buffers are depleted.

Replenishing Balancing Bases

The good news is, you can help your body maintain its delicate pH balance. If you're careful to consume mostly alkaline-forming foods and reduce or eliminate most of the acid-forming ones, you can avoid suffering the symptoms of overacidification and steer clear of much of what has come to be thought of as the natural consequences of aging.

By staying properly hydrated, breathing well, getting adequate (but not excessive) exercise, and consuming foods and beverages with an abundance of alkalizing minerals, you can lessen the likelihood of developing such diseases—and you may be able to reduce or eliminate some of their associated symptoms altogether!

What are those alkaline minerals? Here are the main four:

- Calcium
- Magnesium
- Potassium
- Sodium (not table salt!)

ACID ALERT!

Do not confuse sodium with table salt (sodium chloride). Sodium and potassium are essential minerals that work together to balance fluids in the body. Sodium is essential in the body—and most vegetables provide a good, balanced source of this important salt. But table salt is far too abundant in most modern diets and causes the ideal potassium-to-sodium ratio (2:1) to go awry.

You might think selecting alkaline-forming foods with the right balance of alkaline minerals is difficult, but I'm here to tell you it's not (especially with the recipes in this book!). Almost all naturally occurring fresh vegetables and fruits have the proper balance of minerals—and balance is the important thing.

Some foods, however, contain relatively high concentrations of calcium, magnesium, potassium, and sodium, as you can see in the following table.

Foods High in Alkalizing Minerals

Calcium	Magnesium	Potassium	Sodium
Asparagus	Almonds	Avocados	Avocados
Basil	Broccoli	Bananas	Beets
Broccoli	Brown rice	Beets	Cabbage
Brussels sprouts	Celery	Broccoli	Carrots
Cabbage	Chard	Carrots	Cauliflower
Celery	Cucumbers	Chard	Chile peppers
Chard	Navy beans	Cucumbers	Dark greens (all kinds)
Dark greens (all kinds)	Pumpkin	Dark greens (all kinds)	Eggplant
Garlic	Pumpkin seeds	Kidney beans	Kale
Green beans	Quinoa	Lentils	Lettuce
Kelp	Rice bran	Potatoes (white)	Parsley
Romaine lettuce	Salmon	Soybeans	Radishes

continues

Foods High in Alkalizing Minerals (continued)

Calcium	Magnesium	Potassium	Sodium
Spinach	Soybeans	Spinach	Seaweed
Squash	Spinach	Squash	Sunflower seeds
Thyme	Sunflower seeds	Sweet potatoes	Sweet potatoes
Turnips	Tomatoes	Tomatoes	Turnips

By eating foods rich in alkalizing minerals such as these, your body will restock its reserves and always have plenty on hand to fight imbalance. It will rapidly begin cleansing and detoxifying, rebuilding and replacing old tissues, and repairing past damage.

Soon you'll be astonished at how great you feel!

The Least You Need to Know

- The pH level of the body's various tissues is normally held within very tight bounds. When these levels cannot be consistently maintained, the resulting toxicity gives way to the chronic illness and diseases common to old age.
- The body's elimination organs—especially the kidneys, lungs, and skin—work to expel excessive acids and maintain a slightly alkaline balance in the body.
- When the kidneys, lungs, and skin cannot keep up with the demand for acid elimination, the body draws upon its alkaline reserves, including calcium from the bones.
- By balancing your diet in favor of alkaline-forming foods, you can prevent and correct hyperacidity, bone loss, and many other chronic diseases associated with old age.

Benefits of the pH Balance Diet

In This Chapter

- The standard American diet
- The role pH plays in your body
- Categorizing acidic and alkaline foods
- Weighing benefits against risks
- The findings of Dr. Otto Warburg

Over the past several decades, great medical breakthroughs have been announced and new therapies have been developed, yet the major diseases of our era—cancer, heart disease, and diabetes—remain. Newer diseases such as dementia, osteoporosis, and infertility are gaining ground, too. How can this be?

Rather than looking at the causes of disease, medicine seems more interested in removing the symptoms. With cancer, for example, a typical approach might include surgically removing the tumor and killing problematic cells with chemicals or radiation. But this doesn't prevent or cure cancer. So what's missing from the equation? In a word, *diet*.

In this chapter, we look at the importance of your diet on your health and spotlight what the pH balance diet can do for you.

Your Diet and Your Health

The root cause of so much of modern disease can be found on our dinner plates. The standard American diet (SAD) is at the core of much of the poor state of Americans' health.

PHABULOUS PHACT

The idea that diet is important to overall health isn't new—the Greek physician Hippocrates and ancient Chinese philosophers both recognized it.

No other people in history have eaten the way we do. My grandmother probably wouldn't recognize any of the modern food products routinely advertised today, and she certainly wouldn't recognize much of what's on grocery store shelves. The foods she prepared for her family didn't require labels with lists of ingredients. Artificial additives, flavor enhancers, and chemical preservatives hadn't yet been invented. The only methods of food preservation available to her were drying, canning, brining, and smoking—for many years, she didn't even own a freezer. And so it was for her generation and all the generations of people who came before her.

In Grandma's time, leafy greens, beans, and root vegetables grew in home gardens. Cows produced milk, and that milk was made into curds and buttermilk, alive with thriving bacterial cultures. Fruits and nuts grew on trees planted in the yard. The chickens she ate for dinner had scratched and pecked for live bugs and seeds that morning. The connection between living plants and animals and the food people ate was clear.

The truth is, we've become accustomed to thinking of the chemically altered manufactured products sold in boxes and cans as "food." We don't bat an eye at manufactured sausagelike objects that appear to be meaty hotdogs and yellow curds that resemble freshly scrambled eggs. Using various sophisticated chemical formulas for adding acid-forming artificial flavorings, dyes, and preservatives and neurotoxins like MSG and aspartame, food manufacturers are even able to fool us sometimes. But they don't fool Mother Nature. Manufactured foods aren't the same nurturing, healing sustenance the Earth can give us. We are what we eat. Without *real* food, all living things will eventually become sick and die.

To that, add the fact that most of the food we eat has been cooked, either as part of the manufacturing process itself or as part of meal preparation. According to research conducted in 1930 under the direction of Dr. Paul Kouchakoff in Switzerland, when more than 51 percent of the food we consume is cooked, our bodies enter into a process known as *pathological leukocytosis*. In other words, our bodies treat cooked food as a foreign invader. What do you suppose happens when we eat laboratory engineered products that aren't food at all?

DEFINITION

Pathological leukocytosis is an abnormal condition involving elevated white blood cell counts. It's generally associated with infection, intoxication, poisoning, and consumption of cooked or abnormally altered foods.

If we can't see what happens by examining our own human population, we need look no further than our pet companions. Wild animals eating natural diets don't suffer the debilitating diseases that have become so common among our pet cats and dogs. Like us, our pets are consumers of manufactured food. And just like us, they suffer from chronic and debilitating human disease conditions— cancers, autoimmune disorders, diseases of the liver and pancreas, allergies, obesity, and more.

To prevent or reverse chronic disease, we must find the type of balance in our diets nature intended. pH plays a major role in finding that natural balance.

Your Body and Your pH

Since before World War II, healers from various orthodox and alternative medicine backgrounds have devoted considerable effort to investigating the levels of acidity and alkalinity in the body, and rightfully so. Many vital functions in the body don't occur if not at the proper pH level. For instance, as acidity increases, your muscles' ability to contract declines. At the same time, levels of powerful hormones like adrenaline and aldosterone in your body increase.

The level of pH in the urine or saliva can vary by quite a lot, but your body works hard to keep your blood's pH within tight limits using respiration (breathing), excretion (primarily through the urine and skin), cellular metabolism, and digestion.

When you breathe, for example, your lungs remove carbon dioxide (CO_2) from your body, which aids in acid–alkaline regulation. Red blood cells take the waste product of aerobic respiration (CO_2), convert it to bicarbonate, and release it into the blood. Upon reaching the lungs, it goes back into the red blood cell and is converted back to CO_2 for release in expiration. When the carbon dioxide comes into contact with water in the body, carbonic acid is formed. So with each exhalation, you remove some of this acid as well. Whenever your body's acidity increases, your respiration naturally increases to compensate. As your body becomes more alkaline, your respiration decreases.

Your kidneys play a vital role in maintaining acid–alkaline balance as well. When your blood becomes too acidic, your kidneys help retain sodium and excrete extra hydrogen ions into your urine. This process requires phosphorous, and your body will take phosphorous from your bone tissue if enough isn't available elsewhere. If your body becomes too alkaline, your kidneys will retain hydrogen and release sodium.

ACID ALERT!

When the kidneys aren't functioning properly and begin to fail, the result is a buildup of circulating levels of ammonium ion. Aside from its effect on blood pH, ammonia readily traverses the brain blood barrier and is converted to glutamate in the brain, which depletes the brain of many vital factors. Without these enzymes and other factors, the brain cells can't continue aerobic respiration, and the brain will die.

Digestion also affects your body's pH level. Your stomach secretes hydrochloric acid to break down food. That acid is then absorbed into your bloodstream. To counter the secretion of hydrochloric acid, and to allow another set of digestive enzymes to work, your pancreas secretes alkalizing bicarbonate. The acidity of your blood normally ebbs and flows within a tight margin after eating due to this normal digestive process. This ebb and flow is known as the acid/alkaline tide.

Other digestive events can have a more profound effect on your body's pH. Most notably, diarrhea can cause an increase in acidity, and vomiting causes a decrease in acidity.

When digestive secretions are significantly out of balance, they can have a profound affect on the pH of your entire body. In fact, orthomolecular physician Dr. William Philpott has proposed that cases of severe hyperacidity may be due to the pancreas's inability to secrete sufficient amounts of bicarbonate during the course of normal digestion.

A number of substances exist as components of blood and cellular fluids and various biological processes that also affect the acid–alkaline balance of body tissues. Factors affecting pH balance of the blood include albumin, amino acids, bicarbonate, globulin, and hemoglobin. Chemical reactions that create or consume hydrogen, and hydrogen entering or exiting a cell through diffusion or sodium/potassium pumps, affect the pH of cellular fluids.

Just as your body systems work to regulate their pH levels, individual cells do the same with their own internal pH. One way they accomplish this balancing act is by adjusting internal chemical reactions so fewer hydrogen ions are produced. Another way is through the action of pumps that reside in a cell's membrane. These pumps utilize micronutrient minerals such as magnesium and phosphorus to either take in or expel excess hydrogen.

Acidic and Alkaline Foods

Although the notion of how foods affect the balance of the body's pH levels has been debated for a long time, it's generally accepted that diet is an important source of the alkali and acids your body needs. Yet a debate remains over how to classify acidic and alkaline foods. In general, there are two ways foods have been determined to be acid or alkaline forming.

The first method involves burning foods. When the foods are reduced to their mineral ash counterparts, the pH of the remaining ash is measured and classified according to its level of pH. The following table lists examples of common foods and their classification according to this method of analyzing foods' pH.

Acid, Alkaline, and Neutral Foods—Mineral Ash Method

Acid Ash Foods	Alkaline Ash Foods	Neutral Ash Foods
Brazil nuts and walnuts	Almonds	Arrowroot
Breads and cakes	Cheese	Butter
Cereal grains	Chestnuts	Coffee and tea
Cranberries	Coconut	Cornstarch
Corn	Fruit jams	Lard
Legumes, including peanuts	Milk and cream	Margarine and vegetable oil
Mayonnaise	Molasses	Syrups
Meats	Most fruits	White sugar
Plums and prunes	Most vegetables	Tapioca

The second method considers the various chemical reactions foods ignite within the body. This method reflects what naturopathic practitioners such as Bernard Jensen termed to be acid- or alkaline-forming foods. The following table lists common foods according to whether they're acid or alkaline forming when they're consumed.

Acid-Forming and Alkaline-Forming Foods

Acid-Forming Foods	Alkaline-Forming Foods
All meats, fish and shellfish	All vegetables except legumes (peas, beans, lentils, and peanuts)
All cereal grain foods and products	All fruits except cherries, plums, cranberries, and rhubarb
All fats and oils	Milk
All legumes (peas, beans, lentils, and peanuts)	Buttermilk

Acid-Forming Foods	Alkaline-Forming Foods
All true nuts	Cheese
Chocolate, coffee, and tea	Yogurt
Plant foods containing oxalic acid or benzoic acid: cherries, cranberries, plums, and rhubarb	
Sugar, syrup, and soft drinks	

Many people use the terms *alkaline/acid ash* or *alkaline/acid forming* interchangeably. But as you can see by the preceding tables, these terms don't mean the same things.

Nutritionally speaking, the alkaline ash foods provide greater amounts of alkaline compounds, such as calcium, magnesium, and potassium. Acid ash foods contain minerals that easily form acidic compounds, such as sulfur and phosphorus, or oxalic and benzoic acids that can accumulate in the body's tissues. Trace minerals are an important factor, too. Your kidneys require adequate zinc to excrete or retain acid, as does your stomach when producing acid. Phosphorus and magnesium are required for proper functioning of cellular pumps.

Finally, individual factors determine how foods contribute to your body's pH balance. Certain foods that normally leave no acidic residue may do so in certain individuals, especially those who have low thyroid function or who don't produce adequate amounts of stomach acid for proper digestion. Lifestyle habits also have an impact on the body's pH. Adequate (but not excessive) exercise is alkalizing. Smoking and alcohol use is acidifying.

Those who have championed the pH balance diet recommended an intake of 80 percent alkaline-forming foods to 20 percent acid-forming foods—a ratio of about four vegetables and two fruits to one starch and one protein. On the other hand, important research by Dr. Weston A. Price in the 1930s showed that healthy primitive populations mostly subsisted on acid ash foods, not alkaline ash foods.

The healthiest foods are those that are fresh, nutrient dense, simply prepared, and unrefined.

The Benefits and Risks of a pH Balance Diet

The pH balance diet is thought to be beneficial because it's made primarily of alkalizing vegetables and fruits, augmented by a few soy products, nuts, seeds, legumes, and grains. Proponents of the pH balance diet have claimed everything from the repigmentation of graying hair, weight loss, and decreased pain to cures for cancer, arthritis, and diabetes as a result of following this diet.

In addition, diets high in acid-forming animal fats and proteins have been blamed for countless diseases. Diets made up largely of animal protein, for example, tend to lower the pH of urine, making your body more likely to develop kidney stones and other *ossifications*. According to kidney specialist John Asplin, MD, a pH balance diet that provides an abundance of vegetables lowers risk for developing stones and other kidney disease.

DEFINITION

Ossification is the hardening of soft tissue into bonelike material due to the layering of calcium and other mineral deposits.

Other researchers have theorized that an alkalizing diet might slow bone loss and muscle wasting. The pH balance diet also has been touted as a method of increasing growth hormone production, which, among other things, helps keep you feeling and looking young.

Although there's no direct evidence that a vegetarian or mostly vegetarian diet can prevent cancer, some studies have shown that vegetarians develop cancer at a reduced rate compared to nonvegetarians. No concrete evidence can be established to support this notion, however, because some vegetarians also engage in other practices that lower cancer risk, such as exercising regularly, following stress-reduction routines, and abstaining from alcohol and tobacco products.

Following a pH balance diet that contains optimal levels of fresh vegetables, fruits, grains, and meats is beneficial, if not a cure-all. But there may be a few risks involved in following such a diet.

Diet does not profoundly affect blood pH (because it's mostly self-regulating), and any disturbance in the pH value of blood is an indicator of a serious condition. Uncontrolled blood sugar levels, dehydration, and kidney disease are just three examples.

ACID ALERT!

People with diabetes—especially those who take insulin—and people with kidney disease should never attempt the pH balance diet or any diet without medical supervision.

The Work of Otto Warburg

We're surrounded by a sea of confusing and often contradictory information from different experts about what constitutes a health-promoting/disease-preventing diet.

But as early as 1931, Dr. Otto Warburg published research that showed cancer begins in cells suffering from a lack of oxygen due to weakened cellular respiration. Warburg's research defined and illustrated the environment of cancer cells and showed that these damaged cells begin a type of fermentation process that increases cellular acidity. His work earned him the Nobel Prize.

Cancer

We are aerobic beings—that is, we need oxygen to survive, all the way down to the cellular level. When a cell can no longer "breathe" properly and take in the oxygen required to convert glucose (sugar) into energy, the cell goes to a backup survival plan. In the absence of oxygen, the cell's available sugar begins to ferment, which serves to fuel the cell's energy needs.

Unfortunately, however, this plan works for the short term only. The lactic acid that's the by-product of this fermentation process builds up in and around the cell, lowering its pH. The acidic environment prevents the cell's DNA from controlling normal cell division, and the affected cells begin to multiply wildly. This is cancer.

Dr. Warburg was able to demonstrate that cancer thrives in an acidic, anaerobic environment. He concluded that when the body's tissues can be maintained at a neutral to slightly alkaline level, it's likely that much cancer can be prevented or even reversed. In his lecture, "The Prime Cause and Prevention of Cancer," Warburg stated, "… nobody today can say that one does not know what cancer and its prime cause is. On the contrary, there is no disease whose prime cause is better known, so that today ignorance is no longer an excuse that one cannot do more about prevention." Furthermore, Warburg said, "Cancer, above all other diseases, has countless secondary causes. But even for cancer, there is only one prime cause. Summarized in a few words, the prime cause of cancer is the replacement of the respiration of oxygen in normal body cells by a fermentation of sugar."

BALANCE BONUS

To read "The Prime Cause and Prevention of Cancer," visit healingtools. tripod.com/primecause1.html.

Weight Loss and Blood Pressure

Because of the balance brought about by adding foods rich in alkalizing minerals like potassium to the diet, cells are able to pump fluids in and out at appropriate rates, too. The heart and other muscles are able to contract more efficiently. This facilitates cleansing and detoxification at the cellular level.

When cells are healthy, they tend to release excess fluid. With the loss of fluid retention, natural weight reduction occurs even in the absence of excess body fat, and high blood pressure drops.

Osteoporosis

As mentioned earlier, the blood must be maintained within tight pH bounds. The body uses many strategies to keep the blood's pH in balance, include taking from the bones and other mineral-rich tissues to balance excess acid in the blood. This works out well for the blood but not so well for the tissue.

Chronic hyperacidity is thought to be a major contributor to osteoporosis, muscle wasting, and even poor dental health. By consuming adequate amounts of mineral-rich green leafy vegetables, you can avoid many of the painful and debilitating conditions such as osteoporosis brought on by your body's robbing of your bones to help your blood.

Gout and Arthritis

Gout occurs when you have a buildup of uric acid crystals in your joints. It's a painful condition that, like arthritis, can ultimately be crippling.

By following the pH balance diet and avoiding foods high in uric acid–forming purines, you can slow or even halt the damage done by gout flare-ups. For the most part, high-purine foods are also high-protein foods—organ meats like kidney; fish like mackerel, herring, sardines, and mussels; and yeast. But other otherwise healthy foods can make trouble for gout sufferers as well—dried beans and spinach, in particular.

Cranberries and Other Acid Ash Fruits

Cranberries are an exceptionally healthy food. Although most sources would exclude them because they're an acid ash food, there is room for cranberries in a pH balance diet. Balancing your diet's pH does not mean eating alkalizing foods exclusively—that would be imbalanced in the other direction.

Cranberries contain three acids: quinic, malic, and citric. Their acidity is what researchers once believed made cranberry juice a safe and effective choice for preventing urinary tract infections (UTIs). However, a number of studies and clinical trials have found this isn't quite the case.

Although cranberries contain acidic compounds, they also contain an important phenol compound that's at the crux of their ability to prevent infection. Cranberries and other fruits of shrubs in the genus *Vaccinium*, like blueberries, contain phenol compounds known as *proanthocyanidins*. Proanthocyanindins can inhibit *Escherichia coli* (E. coli) bacteria's ability to attach itself to the lining of the urinary tract, and E. coli is the number-one cause of UTIs. The fructose in cranberries also helps prevent E. coli from attaching to uroepithelial cells that line the interior of the urinary tract.

So while you're concerning yourself with balancing pH, don't avoid all acid ash fruits and vegetables. Although they may contribute to a slight and brief increase in acidity, they also possess many other nutritional factors your body needs.

The Least You Need to Know

- The root cause of many of the symptoms of modern disease is the excessive amount of processed, non-nutritious food in the standard American diet.
- The body needs a proper pH balance to function well.
- Be sure 80 percent of the foods you eat are fresh, natural, and unprocessed.
- The benefits of the pH balance diet outweigh potential risks and include cancer, osteoporosis, and gout prevention; weight loss; and blood pressure management.

Making the pH Balance Diet Work for You

In Part 2, you learn how to monitor your body's pH and adjust your eating and activities to achieve and maintain an optimal pH level. I provide ready-made menu plans, tips on customizing your diet, and easy ways of getting back on track if you find yourself struggling.

In these chapters, you also discover which foods and equipment best help set you up for success. I give you tips on how to shop, prepare, and store fresh fruits and vegetables so they remain fresh longer. You also learn many strategies for keeping your pH balanced while maintaining control in your kitchen.

Finding Your Balance

In This Chapter

- Discovering where your pH stands
- Knowing what your pH readings mean
- Adjusting your diet to suit your particular needs
- Supplementing your diet with green drinks, minerals, and water

If your diet has been a SAD one, you may assume that your body is functioning in a more acidic pH range than is what is ideal. But can you tell for certain whether you are suffering from hyperacidity, and by how much? Yes! The simplest method of doing so is by monitoring the pH value of your urine.

By charting your urine's pH while you make dietary and lifestyle changes, you will have a good indicator of how much progress you're making in your efforts to alkalize. You will also learn which of your changes are having the most impact. This chapter is devoted to teaching you how to test your pH and which foods, supplements, and other strategies can assist you on your journey.

Testing for Balance

The body is constantly making adjustments in order to rid itself of excess acids that cause inflammation of tissues and deplete the body of vital minerals. One of its greatest resources for accomplishing this task is the renal system via the action of the kidneys. Normally, the urine's pH should fall between 7 (neutral) and 7.5 (slightly alkaline). When the pH value of the urine falls below this level, it indicates that the body is using the kidneys to eliminate a greater quantity of acid than normal, which is a sign the body is in a hyperacidic state.

So unlike the blood, which is normally held tightly within safe margins, the pH of urine corresponds closely to the body's internal environment, indicating whether a more or less acidic state exists. By charting your urine's pH, you will gain valuable information about your body's internal environment and how it is metabolizing acids.

Tools of the Trade

The only tools you need to measure urinary pH are litmus test strips. You can buy these in pharmacies, online, and in many health food stores. Litmus test strips are impregnated with a substance that causes them to change color in response to the pH level of moist substances they contact. The color indicates whether the substance is acidic or alkaline in nature, and the intensity of the color indicates the pH's relative strength or weakness.

PHABULOUS PHACT

Litmus paper gets its name from an Old Norse word for lichens that means "to dye." For many centuries, Scandinavians have been using the lichens that provide the dye that gives litmus paper its color to dye cloth.

Each of the possible shades of color on the test strip corresponds to a precise pH value, which is determined by comparing the test strip's results against the various color values on a pH chart that comes as part of the test strip kit. Most litmus test strips allow pH measurements between 4.5 and 9, which is an abundantly broad range for our purposes. Others have a narrower range of between 5.2 and 7.4.

Furthermore, the changes from one shade to the next are indications of half-unit values or less, such as 4.5, 5.0, 5.5, 6.0, and so on. This is helpful in pinpointing minor changes as the urine's pH approaches the neutral pH range. Some brands of pH test strips have unit increments as small as .25. These small increments are helpful in detecting changes when the urine's pH is far from the desired neutral target.

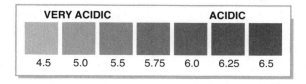

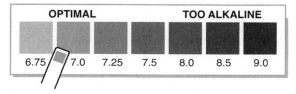

A litmus test strip is matched to the color chart to determine pH value.

All brands I've used have been dependable, so I generally choose the brands that offer the most tests per dollar spent. Some brands are marketed for the express purpose of testing urine to balance the body's pH, and these often are sold together with a package of alkalizing mineral supplements. Check the shelves for similar supplements before deciding to buy pH strip/supplement combination packages because often these combination packages are priced higher than you might pay for each item separately.

Although the appearance and colors used on test strips vary from one brand to another, they all perform the same task equally well. On all varieties of test strips, the color shade indicators change significantly enough from one value to the next that it's generally easy to match the test strip to the proper pH value. For people who have problems with color vision, there are even brands whose test strips have three or more color pads on a single test strip with differing color values, which makes reading them much easier.

Testing for pH

In order to use a litmus pH test strip, you need to expose it to the substance that is being tested. In the case of testing urinary pH, the simplest method of doing this is to quickly pass the test strip through the urinary stream as you urinate—just long enough to dampen it.

The urine will react with the indicators on the strip and cause them to change color according to the level of the urine's pH. You then match the color of the reactive indicator to a corresponding color on the chart that came with your test strips; the number next to that color is the value of your urine's pH. Remember that a neutral pH has a value of 7. Any urine that registers below 6.5 is considered acidic, and a urinary pH above 7.5 is alkaline.

The significance of your urinary pH becomes apparent over time after you have collected a series of data. Just as your internal environment ebbs and flows, your urinary pH varies throughout the day and according to the foods and drink you have consumed, your level of stress, and many other factors. You need to collect and document a minimum of one week's readings, taken at several intervals during the day, before you can draw any significant conclusions.

The first urination of the day contains all the acid that has been eliminated via the kidneys during the course of the night and is much more concentrated than other urinations. For these reasons, it is not used for testing. Urinary pH testing should begin with the second urination of the day and continue with tests *before* eating your noon and evening meals. Testing before meals is important because the foods you eat can significantly skew your results if you test soon after meals. Any additional testing you may choose to do is probably not going to contribute much to your data, but it can be collected and charted nonetheless. You need only a simple notebook to keep track of your pH data.

Be sure to record anything that seems significant to you. Did you go off of your diet plan? Were you unduly stressed that day? Increased demands at work, exercise, drinking too much alcohol or too little water, and illnesses can have a significant impact on your pH—even a day or two after such events have occurred.

After about a week of testing and charting, you'll begin to see a pattern emerge in your pH values. Unless there have been many out-of-the-ordinary occurrences, you can expect your readings to stay relatively consistent from day to day and week to week.

Interpreting Your Test Results

Interpreting your results is not too terribly difficult because pH is defined by only three different possibilities—neutral (7), acidic (below 7), and alkaline (7.5 and above). If your readings are below 7, it indicates that your internal environment is acidic. You can deal with this cut-and-dry matter by beginning a pH balance diet regimen. The lower the reading is, the greater the degree of internal acidification. Any reading below 5 indicates a severe acid imbalance and should be addressed right away.

Most of the time, readings between 7 and 7.5 are ideal. However, it's better if the first urine tested in the morning is on the acidic side. At first this might sound incorrect, but if the first urine tested is either neutral or alkaline and subsequent readings are virtually neutral, your body is not effectively flushing out the night's accumulated acids from the day before. So even if your tests are neutral, if the first test in the morning is not acidic, you have an internally acidic environment. In this condition, your skin and kidneys need some extra help in their work of elimination. Follow the pH balance diet and add dry skin brushing and more hydration to stimulate your kidneys.

If your urinary pH readings are fairly consistently above 7.5 (alkaline), there may be something important amiss. There are four possibilities that must be acknowledged and dealt with.

The first possibility is that your internal environment is in a healthy, slightly alkaline balance. This is especially probable if you are a strict vegetarian who eats plenty of green, leafy vegetables and very little in the way of grains and dairy products. Be happy in the knowledge that your pH is balancing nicely.

ACID ALERT!

Strict vegetarians are at risk for developing nutritional deficiencies, especially in protein and vitamin B_{12}. Be sure you're getting adequate sources of these nutrients in your diet if you're a vegetarian.

Another possibility for why you might consistently have alkaline urinary pH readings would be if you are regularly taking alkalizing mineral supplements when either you don't need them or you need less than what you are accustomed to taking. This situation is not necessarily dangerous, but you should continue to monitor it. If you are taking alkalizing mineral supplements, you may want to reduce your dosage until your urinary pH returns to a more neutral reading.

A third possibility, although extremely rare, is that your pH is consistently alkaline at a level of above 7.5 due to an endocrine abnormality that involves the parathyroid or adrenal glands. People who have such disorders, however, generally are well aware of it and are under a well-supervised treatment plan headed by a physician who specializes in the management of such disorders.

The fourth reason that urine may consistently register in the very alkaline range is that a large amount of alkalizing minerals have been mobilized from the body's tissue stores and dumped into the blood in an effort to buffer an exceedingly acidic internal environment. This environment is usually due to a metabolic defect. People with this defect have difficulty dealing with weak-acid foods. The weak acids in their foods are not properly digested, and the kidneys have a hard time eliminating them. These acids accumulate in the body's tissues until a dangerous level of acidification has been reached.

To protect itself, the body pulls huge quantities of alkaline minerals from its reserves and dumps them into the mix. This process keeps the blood within its acceptable pH range, but causes urine to become very alkaline. Although it seems counterintuitive, the urine has not become alkaline because of the intake of excessive amounts of alkaline minerals, but rather because of the tremendous loss of those same minerals that occurred when the body had to rob its own reserves.

In cases like this, it is imperative to begin alkalizing the diet and using other strategies to bring the internal environment back into balance. When this is accomplished, the urinary pH will begin to drop into a neutral range.

Finally, urinary pH values that are normally inconsistent over the course of each day usually indicate excess internal acidity as well.

Decoding Urinary pH

Average pH of Urine	pH of First Urine	Indicates	Comments	Action
7 or lower (acidic)	7 or lower (acidic)	Acidic internal environment	Created by acidic foods/ lifestyle	Increase alkalizing foods and exercise, manage stress, and hydrate
7 to 7.5 (neutral)	7 or lower (acidic)	Neutral internal environment	If the first urine is acidic, this indicates good pH balance and good general health	Carry on as you have been doing
7 to 7.5 (neutral)	7 to 7.5 (neutral)	Acidic internal environment	If the first urine is also neutral, it indicates the body is not metabolizing acids well	Increase alkalizing foods, exercise, stress management, hydration; practice dry skin brushing
More than 7.5 (alkaline)	7.5 or lower	Alkaline internal environment	Usually due to an exclusively vegetarian diet or too many alkalizing food supplements	Increase protein consumption and/or reduce alkalizing supplements
More than 7.5 (alkaline)	More than 7.5 (alkaline)	Acidic internal environment	Demineralization is being used to buffer excessive acid buildup in the body	Vigorously follow an alkalizing diet; increase alkalizing supplements, hydration, and stress management; decrease protein in diet (beans, grains, and meats)

Classifying Foods

Generally speaking, any of the foods you eat can be classified as either acidifying foods, alkalizing foods, or *weak-acid foods*. Whether a food is acidifying or alkalizing has to do with the effect that digesting that food has on the body. In the case of weak-acid foods, however, it is the food's acid content that is of concern. For some people, a mildly acidic food that would normally have an alkalizing effect is not metabolized correctly, and in those people these weak-acid foods become acidifying in their systems. For those who have difficulty in digesting weak acids, this third way of classifying foods is important.

DEFINITION

Weak-acid foods (mostly tart fruits, whey, and vinegar) have an alkalizing effect on people who properly metabolize weak acids, but are acidifying for people who metabolize acids poorly, if they are able to metabolize them at all. Weak-acid foods are classified as such because they cannot reliably be classified according to the effects (acidifying or alkalizing) they bring about in people.

In the case of people whose bodies are able to metabolize acids properly, the total percentage of alkalizing and weak-acid foods should be greater than the percentage of acidifying foods. On the other hand, if a person has a metabolic inability to handle acids, the percentage of alkalizing foods should always be higher than the total percentage of acidifying and weak-acid foods. And although many people may be able to maintain a healthy acid–alkaline balance while consuming a diet of 50 percent acidifying foods and 50 percent alkalizing foods, people with an acid imbalance should make alkalizing foods 60 to 80 percent of their diet.

As tempting as it might seem for those with an intolerance for weak acids, the idea of eliminating or even severely reducing wholesome acidifying foods is not a wise one. The acidifying foods are usually those that are richest in protein such as eggs, cheese, fish, meats, beans, and grains. The proteins found in acidifying foods are integral to the building and repair of most tissues in the body. Furthermore, they form a sort of matrix for holding minerals in our tissues. Without adequate protein intake, many of the minerals we consume would not establish themselves in our tissues to be available for neutralizing acids, but would be flushed away, so to speak.

So it is important to vary your foods while keeping in mind that the more acidic a person's internal environment is, the more important it is to consume plenty of alkaline foods with every meal. These foods help to alkalize the other foods you consume, without the need for drawing on the body's mineral reserves.

The pH balance diet is a corrective diet by nature. Most people can follow a pH balance diet plan like the one in Chapter 5 and observe immediate benefits and an improvement in their sense of well-being. For those who are on the metabolic fringe, however—unable to metabolize weak acids, as evidenced by extremes in pH urine data— the following lists can help in determining how to push forward with further diet adjustments.

Acidifying Foods

If you are having difficulty obtaining a consistently balanced pH reading, the following foods may be part of the problem. Although no particular food is forbidden on a pH balance diet, the effects of consuming some foods pose no problem for some people, yet they cause great difficulty for others. The most problematic foods are those that are acidifying, which include the following:

- Meat of all kinds: sausages, cold cuts, bouillon, shellfish, fish, poultry, beef, pork, lamb, and so on.
- Other animal fats and proteins, such as eggs, lard, suet, and hard cheeses
- Refined vegetable oils and all hydrogenated oils, such as margarines and shortening
- Refined or whole grains (except corn) and grain-based foods—especially wheat and millet—including breads, cakes, noodles, pasta, crackers, cereals, and breading
- Beans and legumes, including soybeans and peanuts
- Sugars, syrups, and candies

- Fruit jams, jellies, and preserves
- Coffee, caffeinated teas, spirits, wine, beer, and soft drinks
- Common salad and sandwich condiments, such as mustard, mayonnaise, ketchup, and commercially prepared dressings
- Oily nuts and seeds such as walnuts and pumpkin seeds—*but not* coconut, Brazil nuts, or almonds

Weak-Acid Foods

As explained earlier in this chapter, the second group of foods that may be limiting your expected results are the weak-acid foods. Most of these foods normally act in an alkalizing manner, but because of the acids they contain, they can make problems for people who do not metabolize acids well. The following weak-acid foods are commonly eaten:

- Mild soft cheeses like small-curd cottage cheese, yogurt, whey, and kefir
- Acidic fruit such as citrus fruits, tart berries, apples, cherries, apricots, and plums
- Acidic vegetables such as rhubarb and *nightshades* like eggplant, chiles, and tomatoes
- Lacto-fermented products like sauerkraut, natural buttermilk, brined pickles, and cornichons
- Unripened fruits of all kinds
- Honey, fruit juices, and vinegars

DEFINITION

Nightshades are a group of plants that contain powerful alkaloids, some of which are used in prescription medications. A nightshade's alkaloids can impact nerve–muscle function and digestive function and may also be able to compromise joint function. Many nightshades are also strong allergens. Notable nightshades include potatoes, tomatoes, sweet and hot peppers, eggplant, tomatillos, tamarios, pepinos, pimentos, paprika, tobacco, and belladona.

Alkalizing Foods

Alkalizing foods do not contain acids that people with acid-averse metabolic disorders find problematic, and they do not leave an acid ash residue behind as a result of digestion. They are also chock-full of alkalizing minerals that help to buffer your tissues' pH. The alkalizing foods are primarily brightly colored vegetables and leafy greens. These foods should be included at every meal, but especially if you are having difficulty maintaining consistently balanced pH readings. The more out of whack your readings are, the more alkalizing foods you should eat with every meal. Alkalizing foods include the following:

- Pure mineral water
- Leafy green vegetables of all kinds, including lettuces, cabbage, collards, dandelion greens, kale, and a variety of salad greens
- White potatoes—Idaho, russet, and so on
- Chestnuts, almonds, coconut, Brazil nuts, and their natural, cold-pressed oils
- Ripe bananas and avocados
- Dried fruits such as raisins and dates—*but not* those that are tart, such as pineapple and apricots
- Brightly colored vegetables such as carrots, broccoli, and beets, *but not* tomatoes and chiles
- Almond milk, dairy milk, cream, butter, and large-curd cottage cheese
- Corn, corn grits, and polenta
- Black olives preserved in olive oil, *but not* green olives and not olives preserved in vinegar

Alkalizing Supplements

Aside from the food you eat and the water you drink, there is still more that you can do to balance your pH. In fact, there is more that you must do—at least, in the beginning. When you adhere to an alkalizing diet, you are not adding acids or creating new acidic residues that burden the body. But you still have a residual acid burden in your tissues that will take some time and extra effort to clear.

Your kidneys, skin, and lungs can rid the body of only so much acid at a time. As has been mentioned, the blood's pH must stay within tight bounds. Yet in order to clear acids through respiration or excretion, those acids must first be allowed to circulate in the blood. It follows that if too much acid is released from tissues at once, those acids would tip the balance of the blood's pH and a crisis would ensue.

Those acids that the body cannot immediately rid itself of through respiration or excretion are stored in tissues until enough alkalizing minerals have been consumed. Slowly but surely, the acidity of your tissues would begin to resolve and move ever closer to a neutral pH if you followed an alkalizing diet. But you should not and cannot consume only alkalizing foods over the long term. Doing so would mean sacrificing far too many important amino acids, vitamins, and protein. The answer to this conundrum is to take alkalizing supplements while following a pH balance diet.

Green Drinks

One of the most natural ways of introducing a large amount of properly proportioned alkalizing minerals into the diet is by consuming green drinks. Juiced wheatgrass and barley grass are two excellent sources of alkalizing minerals, and I highly recommend them. Just 1 or 2 ounces per day can have quite an astounding impact on how quickly your body can remove acid residues. Most people find that juiced wheatgrass has a sickeningly sweet flavor—saccharine comes to mind—while barley grass is bitter. I like to juice them together, half-and-half, so that their flavors balance one another. There is no good reason to linger and sip the stuff, though, so most people will take a shot of this green juice in the same manner they would a shot of whiskey. Quick and neat.

If you are not interested in growing and juicing your own wheat or barley grass, there are excellent powdered drink mixes that provide the same benefits. One that I would recommend, solely due to my personal experience with it, is Kyo-Green, but many other excellent products are available—Green Vibrance, Barlean's Greens, and ORAC-Energy Greens, to name but a few. In general, these products provide naturally balanced alkalizing minerals from sources like wheat and barley grass, brown rice, kelp, and chlorella. They are easily prepared and don't require juicing equipment. Just 1 teaspoon of these pleasant-tasting powders added to plain water or a smoothie or even sprinkled over food provides great benefits for very little trouble.

BALANCE BONUS

When you buy green drink supplements, you may notice that the label claims to provide a certain level of ORAC. ORAC stands for oxygen radical absorbance capacity. It is a relative measure of the free radical–destroying potential of a particular food. When all other things are equal, always choose a product with the higher ORAC value.

Alkalizing Mineral Supplements

To maintain both health and proper pH, the body needs these five essential minerals:

- Calcium (Ca)
- Potassium (K)
- Magnesium (Mg)
- Iron (Fe)
- Manganese (Mn)

If these minerals are to be of benefit, however, they must be consumed in proper proportion to one another, as well as in proper proportion to their counter-balancing minerals. With minerals, balance is key. So it would be a potentially dangerous mistake to rush out and buy a bottle of potassium capsules and a separate bottle of calcium tablets and begin taking these minerals haphazardly. If you're interested in speeding up the process of buffering stored acids so that they can be safely removed from the body, balanced mineral supplements are available that have been expertly designed to accomplish this.

Ingredients and Attributes of Various Alkalizing Supplements

Product	Calcium	Potassium	Magnesium	Iron	Manganese	Other	Flavor	Tablet	Powdered
Rebasit*	X	X	X	X	X	Sodium and silicon	Savory		X
Ideal Base Plus	X	X	X	X	X	Vitamins B_1, B_2, B_3, B_6, inositol, sodium, and zinc	Savory	X	X
Erbasit	X	X	X	X	X	Elder extract	Citrus	X	X
Alcabase	X	X	X	X	X	Sodium	Savory or citrus	X	X
Basa Vita**	X	X	X	X	X	Whey and silicon	Orange		X
pHion Blue**	X	X	X	X	X	Phosphorus	Citrus	X	X
Basin	X	X	X	X	X	Sodium	Savory		X
Flugge's	X	X	X		X	Sodium and silicon	Savory		X
Alkala	X	X		X	X		Savory		X
Megabase	X	X	X			Anise, absinthe, charcoal, sodium, and silicon	Licorice		X

Contains a relatively large amount of sodium. Not suitable for people with high blood pressure, fluid retention, edema, or heart or kidney disorders.

**Contains no sodium.*

The supplements listed in the preceding table are but a small sampling of those that are available, and most of the products I have found are well balanced and effective. Not everyone has the same needs, though, so it is wise to study the ingredients to be sure that you are not supplementing with a product that provides substances you should avoid. Iron, for instance, would be an element that doctors might recommend cancer patients steer clear of, and sodium should be avoided by people with a variety of other medical conditions.

Along the same lines, because everyone has slightly different needs and conditions, these supplements should be eased into gradually in order to determine the proper amount and duration of dosage. To gain the maximum benefit of alkalizing supplements, you need to take as much as is necessary to bring your urine's pH level into the 7 to 7.5 range consistently.

For instance, if your urine is registering as acidic throughout the day, you might begin by taking a single tablet or a teaspoon of supplement powder with water prior to eating each of your main meals. The next day, if your urine is less acidic, but still not in the 7 to 7.5 pH range, increase your dosage to $1\frac{1}{2}$ teaspoons before meals. Continue in this way, making slight increases in dosage, until your urine consistently falls into the desired slightly alkaline range.

For people who have a high saturation of acids in their tissues, several teaspoons per meal may be required for a time. Because these preparations are well balanced, there is no need for concern about how much is required. If your urine has not come into the desired pH range, your body is telling you it needs this supplementation. On the other hand, once you determine the proper dosage according to the consistently good urinary pH readings, it is no longer necessary to test for pH daily. Testing on two consecutive days per month is sufficient to let you know whether you are still on track or need to make a small adjustment.

Eventually, your urinary pH will rise to a more alkaline level and you will begin to taper off on your regular dosage amounts. This may take six months, a year, or even two years. It all depends on how much your body has been storing acid deposits deep within your tissues. Considering that you might have been building up these acid residues for many decades, even two years is not a long time to have to supplement with the minerals your body needs.

Alkalizing Water

Plain water, on its own, is infinitely helpful in reducing the body's acid load. Pure mineral water is even better. Most proponents of the pH balance diet recommend drinking, at minimum, $\frac{1}{2}$ ounce water for every 1 pound you weigh, daily. For instance, if you weigh 150 pounds, then over the course of a day, you would drink 75 ounces of water.

Some companies, however, sell water ionizers touted to speed up the process of balancing your pH beyond what can be accomplished by drinking pure water. Many alkaline water enthusiasts are convinced the benefits of using this technology are unparalleled and vehemently defend them. But according to natural wellness expert Dr. Joseph Mercola, the claims of health benefits provided by these systems are, at best, unjustified: "… the scientific justification for these water systems is absent and … consumers have merely fallen under the spell of a skilled marketer who selectively misused pseudoscientific information and twisted it around to scare them into buying their product."

Very few legitimate scientific studies about the effects of alkaline water on human health actually exist.

ACID ALERT!

Most water ionizers and alkalizers are marketed using a multilevel marketing (MLM) model that has been known to produce less than ethical results in recent years. The way this works is that a buyer is sold an expensive machine, but the seller will give the buyer a steep discount if he signs up as a representative for the company. The buyer then has a vested interest, as a member of the MLM company, and is likely to continue to push the product even if it is not providing the promised benefits.

On that note, remember that there is no particular product that you must have in order successfully balance your body's pH. Never allow yourself to feel pressured into buying a particular product. Water alkalizers and ionizers may or may not help. They may start out to be helpful and then later deliver fewer benefits. One alkalizing supplement may work better for you than it does for your neighbor, and another supplement might not be a good one for you at all. We are all different and have differing needs that change over time. In the end, the best advice is to keep things simple—in both the foods you eat and the tools you employ.

The Least You Need to Know

- Urinary pH is a good indicator of the condition of the body's internal environment. A week's worth of pH test data must be collected and charted for the readings to reveal any significant meaning.

- High urinary pH readings don't necessarily mean your body's internal environment is alkaline. In fact, consistently alkaline pH results usually mean the opposite.

- It is unwise to eliminate or even strictly reduce high-protein acidifying foods over the long term. These foods are necessary for their nutrient contents and for helping the body's tissues retain alkalizing minerals.

- Do not be duped by people who would have you believe that you must purchase a particular product in order to successfully balance your pH. The pH balance diet is simple and does not require fancy equipment.

Preparing for the pH Balance Diet

In This Chapter

- Assessing where you are now
- Mapping out your goals
- Balancing your kitchen
- Choosing tools that make a difference

Before you launch headlong into your new pH adventure, you need to assess where your diet currently stands, and the foods and tools you have on hand. Doing so helps you form a realistic idea of why you may have been feeling poorly and of how much improvement you can expect.

This chapter helps you clear out the clutter and define a course of action for implementing your personal pH balance diet plan. It also introduces you to some fun kitchen gadgets to assist you in the new methods of food preparation that await. If you're a consummate foodie like me, you'll be fascinated by what you discover, and you are bound to have lots of fun.

Is Your Diet SAD?

The SAD, or standard American diet, has become an unhealthy way of eating among most Americans. Yet most people are convinced that they eat a fairly healthy diet. And why not? If you really believed what you were eating was toxic or harming your health in some way, you probably would have stopped eating it by now, wouldn't you? But if you ever feel bloated, jittery, or moody; have overwhelming food cravings; or experience low energy, insomnia, or brain fog, you might have your diet to blame—at least to some degree.

The all-important first step in determining whether your diet may be contributing to your health problems, and how much a corrective diet can bring improvement, is to examine your diet exactly as it is now. Without making any changes, you must be honest about everything you eat and drink by keeping a food journal for one week. Once you have the facts about where you're starting from, you can build a road map for improvement.

Your Seven-Day Food Journal

Many people feel they never eat anything. They chronically skip meals. They nibble on something at their desks or during their commute because they feel too busy to stop work. But because they are busy with other tasks, they eat mindlessly, and they are often eating far more (and worse) food than they imagine. To put an end to the ignorance that can surround how much and what kinds of food you may be consuming, you need to become aware of what you're *really* eating.

For this exercise, you need a notebook, a new document on your computer or tablet, or a new note on your smartphone. It doesn't have to be fancy. In fact, low-tech is probably better because your food journal must be with you and accessible at all times.

For one week, record everything you eat and drink—*everything*. Be brutally honest about it. Whether you skipped all meals during a day, or you ate five chocolate bars, pretending it didn't happen by not recording it is not only dishonest, it also hinders you from reaching your goal of becoming the healthiest version of you.

The more specific and detailed you make your journal, the more it will tell you about how and where you can improve. Don't take half-measures in recording your food. For instance, if you had coffee, record when, how many cups, and how much cream and sugar went with it. Was it real cream or nondairy creamer? If you drank water, was it mineral water or plain? If you ate a hamburger, did it have a brand name (such as the Double Bacon Monster Chef with Cheese) or was it homemade? Was it fried or broiled? What did you put on it? Was it open-faced or on a bun? What kind of bun? You get the picture.

BALANCE BONUS

One way to make sure that you are accurately recording what you eat is to save the labels and packaging of the foods you eat. Collect these for a week in a grocery sack. If you eat something fresh, like an apple or cucumber, write that down on a slip of paper and toss it in the sack. Or take photos of the package and nutrition label or fresh item and keep a file on your computer or smartphone of everything that passed your lips. A week's collection of food labels or pictures provides concrete evidence reflecting the state of your nutrition.

Also record in your journal any exercise you may do, both the time and the activity. Did you take a 30-minute walk after work? Did you do heavy gardening on Saturday? Maybe you're a writer and the most activity you had was coaxing words from your brain into your computer via keystrokes. Whatever the physical activity was (or wasn't), write it down.

Additionally, keep track of how you are sleeping. What time did you go to bed? Did you fall asleep right away? Was your sleep fitful? Did you awaken feeling rested in the morning? Were you in so much pain you could hardly roll out of bed?

Finally, observe how you feel before and after eating. You might feel just fine. But you also might feel tired, headachy, or jittery. Don't look at this so critically that you begin to think you might be imagining something that is not there. Simply observe how you feel, and if anything seems to stand out, write it down along with the time you noticed it.

Sample Journal Entry

Monday

5:30 A.M.	2 cups caffeinated black coffee. Woke tired. Had nightmares all night.
8 A.M.	1 glazed doughnut from snack cart. 1 black coffee.
10 A.M.	$\frac{1}{2}$ liter plain bottled water. Still hungry.
12 P.M.	Homemade tuna salad sandwich on whole wheat. 1 small bag barbecue corn chips. 12 ounces diet cola. $\frac{1}{2}$ banana.
2:30 P.M.	12 ounces diet root beer. Feeling sleepy.
3 P.M.	So frustrated with my job. Need something sweet. 1 chocolate bar.
4 P.M.	Ate handful of M&M's.
5:30 P.M.	Drive home. Feeling exhausted.
6 P.M.	1 double mixed drink to wind down.
6:30 P.M.	15-minute walk with the dog.
7:30 P.M.	6-ounce rib-eye steak, grilled. 1 small baked potato with butter, sour cream, and chives. $\frac{1}{2}$ cup steamed broccoli. 3 glasses dry red wine. Small slice deli cheesecake for dessert. Feeling much better.
9 P.M.	So sleepy, can't keep eyes open; going to bed.

By the end of the week, you will notice that some patterns have emerged. It may be that you are eating the same foods all of the time. You may see that you are gravitating to things that you know you should avoid, such as foods that you are allergic to, sugary foods, or alcohol. That's okay, though. This exercise is about acknowledging exactly where you are in relation to your food, and it is the beginning of being able to recognize how and where you can improve.

Your Food Review

After keeping a detailed journal and recording everything you eat either with labels or photos for a week, you need to take a look at what's really been going on in your diet. As you sift through your information, you may be happily surprised—or you might be slightly horrified. But either way, there is no better, more direct route to improving your health than by staring the facts squarely in the face. So take courage and forge ahead. Knowledge is power, and you have all the tedium behind you now.

Review the food labels or photos and your journal. What's the ratio of prepared foods to fresh foods? Take a look at the ingredients labels and begin to familiarize yourself with what's in the food you've been eating. The ingredients on food labels are arranged from beginning to end in the order of their major components, by weight. Is sugar near the top of many of the lists? What about salt? Then there are all those other ingredients—the additives, preservatives, dyes, artificial flavors, enhancers, emulsifiers, and fortifiers. Are these lists long? Are they even pronounceable? All these substances increase the body's toxic load and, therefore, increase acidity, affecting pH by varying degrees.

> **PHABULOUS PHACT**
>
> Of the more than 14,000 chemicals that are added to foods, some of the most common include the preservatives BHA and BHT; monosodium glutamate (MSG), a neurological excitotoxin sometimes referred to as "natural flavor"; nitrates and nitrites; sulfates and sulfites; dyes; artificial flavors; caffeine; and aspartame, phenylalanine (neurotoxins), and other artificial sweeteners.

None of these additives are real food. After keeping a food journal, many people are surprised to discover that they've really been eating quite a lot, but whatever it is they've been eating is not actually food. If you need to look up an ingredient on the internet to learn what it is, it does not belong in a pH balance diet—or any healthy diet, for that matter.

Your Food Profile

Now that you have your food information and journal at hand, turn to Appendix D to create your personal food profile. It will be your map and inspiration on your journey to the optimally balanced diet for you.

Be sure to take your time doing this. There is no rush. You have all the tools you need right in front of you and the desire to fuel your success inside. Read the questions and respond with honest answers, and your road map and personal dietary profile will begin to emerge.

When you're done, you'll be ready to assess the pH of your kitchen, and you will have the additional motivation to make some positive changes there, too.

The pH Balance of Your Kitchen

What's in your pantry? You probably think you know, but now it's time to take a real inventory. If you've been following a SAD diet, the pH balance of your kitchen is probably in need of a little adjustment. Assessing what your pantry, refrigerator, and freezer hold can be a rewarding and eye-opening experience.

For many people, however, this second step in transitioning to an alkaline diet is the scariest part. But don't let it frighten you. If at the end of your pantry reconnoiter you find you have to toss more food than you keep, count it a good day! Take the opportunity to wipe down your now near-empty cupboards to prepare for the new foods and improved health that lie ahead for you. It's cause to celebrate!

Toss the Forbidden Foods

The comprehensive food tables in Appendix C should be your guides when deciding whether a particular food should stay or go. But just so there's no confusion, clear out all of the following from your diet for at least the next 28 days:

- Alcohol (wine coolers, beer, wine, spirits)
- Caffeinated drinks (coffee, black tea, colas, sports/energy drinks)
- Cakes, cookies, and pastries
- Canned foods with additives, sugar, or salt
- Carbonated drinks and powdered drink mixes
- Candy, chocolate, and chewing gum
- Cow's milk, hard cheeses, and ice cream

- Chips and pretzels
- Frozen or ready-made meals
- Frozen pizza
- Margarine
- Packaged foods with additives, sugar, or salt
- Processed meats (lunchmeat, sausages, bacon, ham, and so on)
- Red meat
- Sugar and syrups
- Table salt
- Wheat products (flour, bread, biscuits, crackers, pasta, and so on)
- White rice

As I mentioned in Chapter 3, there really are no "forbidden" foods in a pH balance diet. But for the time being, and in order to experience what it feels like when you are eating in a balanced manner, these items need to go. If you spend the next 28 days diligently following the pH balance diet, you will probably notice such an improvement in how you feel that you won't miss the food you tossed out.

On the other hand, if there is a slip here or there, you will still improve. This diet is about working toward balance, and any improvements move you in the direction of achieving that balance.

BALANCE BONUS

Whenever you are hungry, or if you begin to have food cravings, you can always eat fresh fruits and vegetables until you are satisfied. Additionally, you can treat yourself to any of the great smoothies in Chapter 8, make yourself a huge glass of fresh vegetable juice, or even enjoy a comforting and filling bowl of soup. And don't forget—this book even has some scrumptious desserts!

Restock Your Shelves

Do you feel like Old Mother Hubbard now? Are your cupboards all bare? They won't be for long!

When you looked at your food journal, did you notice any patterns? You should see patterns in the times of day you eat, and in the times of day you choose to eat or drink certain types of things. Most people's daily routines have a rhythm to them. I bet that there is also a remarkable similarity in the kinds of foods you choose to eat day after day. If you kept a food journal for a whole month, you would see that, for the most part, you are choosing to eat the same 10 or 15 foods over and over again!

Sometimes food preference is a cultural thing. For instance, in a Cajun household, the average evening fare would almost certainly include "rice and gravy." It's so pervasive, you can hardly pronounce the one word without the other. The name of this dish also implies that red meat is served along with it because that is where the gravy comes from. Along with the meat and rice and gravy, one or two vegetables and a modest salad would form an average traditional Cajun meal.

You might think the vegetables and salad would allow for some variety. They certainly do. But people get stuck in ruts. In some families, salad might mean coleslaw or potato salad and is served repeatedly because Suzy doesn't like lettuce, Mary is allergic to tomatoes, and Dad thinks fresh carrots and spinach are rabbit food. This same family's vegetables might consist of a rotation of corn, green beans, and sweet peas because those are what the grocer usually has on sale.

This is a "sad" diet of a different kind. There is nothing inherently wrong with it, except for the fact that there is little or no variety. Your body deserves better than the same 10 or 15 foods *ad nauseam* when nature's bounty provides so much more!

For the next 28 days, your goal is to eat like a king. You don't have to count calories, fat grams, carbohydrates, or portions. Just don't eat any of the foods you just tossed out. In their place, you'll enjoy foods that will surprise and delight your palate. Although you gave the boot to nearly everything in your pantry, you still can have so much, as the following table shows.

Permissible Foods on an Alkalizing Diet

Fish	Greens	Vegetables	Grains
Cod	Arugula	Acorn squash	Amaranth
Flounder	Chard	Artichokes	Barley
Haddock	Cress	Avocados	Brown rice
Herring	Dandelion	Beets	Buckwheat
Mackerel	Endive	Bok choy	Kamut
Monkfish	Escarole	Broccoli	Oats
Pollack	Kale	Carrots	Quinoa
Salmon	Mustard	Cassava	Red rice
Sardines	Romaine	Cauliflower	Spelt
Sea bass	Sorrell	Celeriac	Teff
Snapper	Spinach	Eggplant	Rye
Trout	Turnips	Fennel	Wild rice

And this is just the short list! In addition to the exhaustive list of wonderful fish, greens, veggies, and grains in Appendix C, you will find a mind-boggling variety of beans, sprouts, seeds, and nuts. There are sea vegetables, alternative flours, herbs, fruits, melons, and teas, too. Believe it or not, even chicken, turkey, tofu, and yogurt are not off limits.

Tools of the Trade

Many people I meet think cooking means opening a few packages, stirring in some water, and heating it all up on the stove or in the microwave oven. These people will try to chop onions with a steak knife because they don't know any better. Because they lack the proper tools, they are easily discouraged and find food preparation daunting. Don't let that be you.

A few wonderful tools can make food preparation a joy. Nearly none of them are absolutely necessary, but the right tools can make all the difference when you are cooking—and the pH balance diet requires a little real cooking.

Cut Up in the Kitchen

Number one on my list of must-haves is the right knife. Whether you opt for a butcher knife, a French chef's knife, or a Japanese cleaver, the important thing is to select a knife that will serve you well and that you're comfortable using. Without a good knife, there is little you can accomplish with food. With the *right* knife, you can do almost everything. It may take a little shopping around to find the right knife for you, but the effort and any related expense are well worth it.

My favorite knife is a carbon steel Old Hickory butcher knife. It measures $12\frac{1}{2}$ inches from tip to tang and boasts a mighty $8\frac{1}{4}$-inch blade and a replaceable riveted wooden handle. With it, I can peel a grape, slice a tomato, dice an onion, smash and mince a clove of garlic, or dispatch a side of beef. And it does not tire my wrist or hand.

Consider getting these other helpful cutting gadgets as well:

- Food processor
- *Mandoline*
- *Spiralizer*
- Zester
- Vegetable peeler

DEFINITION

A **mandoline** is a classic French food prep tool used for uniformly slicing firm vegetables. With suitable attachments, it can make julienne, crinkle, and waffle cuts as well. A **spiralizer** is a simple, lathelike cutting tool that can fashion spaghetti or flat noodle shapes from raw zucchini, carrots, and other vegetables.

Bring on the Juice!

Another important piece of equipment to have is a juicer. In a pH balance diet, you will drink freshly made vegetable juices every day. So unless you live next to a 24-hour juice bar, you will need to borrow or own a juicer.

Almost any juicer will do a good job for you, and juicers are available in a wide range of prices and features. I own both a slow-speed, single-auger juicer and a high-speed, centrifugal juicer, and I am pleased with them both.

My favorite is the auger-style juicer, though. It does a great job of juicing wheatgrass and leafy greens—the high-speed juicer does not. The slow-speed, single-auger juicer will juice vegetables and fruits, too, and it can be used for making nut butters and gazpacho-style soups. Additionally, because of the auger's slow turning speed, the juice does not heat up during processing. This means that the juice does not undergo much oxidative stress and remains fresher longer.

Take It Slow

Do you have a slow cooker? (Or three, like my editor?) Nothing compares to the tremendous nutrition and deeply satisfying comfort provided by slow-cooked homemade soups and stews. Also, no other method of cooking beans is as foolproof. Plus, a slow cooker frees you to do other things while it does all the work.

After minimal preparation, you set the ingredients in the crock, cover it, turn it on, and forget about it for 6 to 12 hours. Easy! Also, it doesn't heat up your kitchen, and it doesn't cook so hot that vitamins are obliterated. There is no roiling steam through which nutrition can escape.

Other Handy Gadgets

The following tools recommended for your pH balance kitchen are geared more toward speed and ease than anything else:

- Handheld immersion blender
- Stainless-steel pressure cooker
- Salad spinner
- Mortar and pestle

The immersion blender, or blender wand, is handy for making whole-grain creamed cereals, puréed soups, smooth sauces, and salad dressings in a jiffy—and it cleans up just as quickly. Simply unscrew the business end, rinse, and rack dry.

Anything you can cook on the stovetop will cook faster in a pressure cooker and use less energy, too. Pressure cookers are wonderful for cooking brown rice, beans, and stews on short notice.

> **ACID ALERT!**
>
> Do not use aluminum cookware or nonstick, Teflon-coated pans. Aluminum leaches out of cookware into your food, and it has been associated with neurodegenerative diseases. DuPont's studies show that, at cooking temperatures, Teflon pans "release at least six toxic gases, including two carcinogens, two global pollutants, and MFA, a chemical lethal to humans at low doses," writes Jane Houlihan in *Canaries in the Kitchen: Teflon Toxicosis*. Better choices include cast iron, stainless steel, glass, and earthenware.

Salad spinners are inexpensive little wonders that dry off your washed salad greens so that salad dressing will stay on the salad where it belongs instead of on the bottom of the salad bowl. They also make marvelously entertaining toys for little ones who want to visit with you in the kitchen as you perform your pH magic.

Finally, the utility of a natural stone mortar and pestle cannot be beat. From bruising fresh herbs to grinding small quantities of seeds and spices, nothing else gets the job done in such a simple way.

Over time, you might want to add a bamboo steamer, a food dehydrator, a rice or grain cooker, an electric spice or coffee mill, and sprouting jars or bags to your pH balance kitchen.

Principles of Proper Food Combining

Food combining is an approach to eating that eases the body's job of digesting foods and therefore results in less acid production. It is based on the premise that certain foods must remain in the stomach to be broken down far longer than other foods. If these foods are eaten at the same time with foods that break down more rapidly, the fast-digesting foods will begin to ferment and putrefy before they are released into the small intestine. This process does not make for good nutrition or proper pH. If you ever have flatulence, indigestion, heartburn, or other stomach upsets, proper food combining is highly recommended as a preventative measure. Additionally, water and other liquids should not be ingested too close to mealtime.

Quick Guide to Proper Food Combining

Best Eaten on an Empty Stomach	Eat with Cooked, Nonstarchy Vegetables	Eat with Cooked, Nonstarchy Vegetables	Eat with Raw Vegetables	Combines Well with Any Other Foods
Apples	Avocados	Cheese	Bananas	Almond milk
Avocados	Bread	Eggs	Dried fruit	Butter
Bananas	Grains	Fish	Nuts	Coconut water
Berries	Noodles	Milk	Seeds	Lemons
Cherries	Pasta	Meat		Limes
Mangoes	Potatoes			Unrefined oils
Melons	Young coconut meat			Unsweetened chocolate
Papayas	Winter squash			Raw, leafy greens
Any other fruits	Beans and legumes			

Now that you have assessed your old diet and the tools you have on hand, you are ready to get started. You've done a lot of hard work and you deserve to be congratulated—I hope you feel inspired! The clutter has been cleared from your larder, and you have pinpointed areas in your lifestyle that you want to improve. The only thing left is to check out your shopping lists in Chapter 5 and get started!

The Least You Need to Know

- Honest evaluation of your current eating habits will help you to identify changes that you may need to make and will highlight your healthy dietary goals.

- Your goals and dietary plan are personal with respect to you. You already have all the answers before you and inside of you to make your pH transition a smashing success.

- The pH balance diet may change the types of foods you eat, but you can eat without ever counting calories, carbohydrates, or fat grams.

- Collecting the right food prep tools and equipment can mean all the difference in how much you enjoy your pH balance diet experience.

pH Balance Menu Plans

In This Chapter

- Expanding your menu options
- Planning simple and easy menus
- Tips for getting back on track

In this chapter, you put your newly gained knowledge into practice with menus for beginning and succeeding with the pH balance diet. As you become familiar with some of the new foods and flavor possibilities, you'll soon be confidently selecting the meals and snacks you enjoy the most.

A Few Notes

The following menus might call for foods you're allergic to. If that's the case, substitute that food with one you can safely eat.

Sometimes you won't be able to find every food on the menu. That's no problem. Just substitute something else. If no good substitute is available, leave out the ingredient. These recipes are forgiving.

If one apple is suggested as a snack, or a serving size is listed as 1 cup, there's nothing to stop you from eating two apples or more than 1 cup instead. This diet is mostly good-for-you raw fruits and vegetables, so the more you get, the better! Just eat slowly so you can recognize when you're full.

Throughout the pH balance diet, you'll be drinking herbal teas that possess many health-promoting benefits, and a variety of teas are available. Sage tea, for example, is a calming liver and kidney tonic, helpful for alleviating joint pain and a sore throat. Dandelion tea is helpful in maintaining optimum liver, kidney, and gallbladder function; enhances detoxification by stimulating urination; and replaces the potassium lost to the increased volume of urine. It supports healthy blood sugar levels and good digestion and helps purify and cleanse the blood. Nettle tea helps relieve coughs and asthma; muscle, joint, and tendon pain; and allergic eczema and hay fever. It's also helpful in the prevention of urinary tract infections.

Week 1

This week will probably be the most trying one for you. Please try to eat the suggested foods in good faith—especially those new to you. They may taste unusual at first, but as your body begins to cleanse and adjust, you'll discover some tasty new favorites!

Day 1

Greet the day with a tall glass of water and a squeeze of lemon.

Breakfast: Quick Oats (Chapter 9) sprinkled with cinnamon, raisins, and chopped walnuts; Sunrise Smoothie (Chapter 8) or sage tea with lemon and honey (optional)

Morning snack: 2 or 3 celery ribs

Lunch: Cut raw vegetables, Wholly Guacamole (Chapter 12), Hippocrates Soup (Chapter 14), large mixed-greens salad with your choice dressing (Chapter 11; optional)

Afternoon snack: Raw almonds

Dinner: Sweet Potato, Chipotle, and Kidney Bean Chili (Chapter 14); cooked brown rice; steamed spinach

Evening snack: 1 or 2 apples

Day 2

Greet the day with a tall glass of water and a squeeze of lemon.

Breakfast: Savory Quinoa Breakfast Bowl (Chapter 9), Basic Strawberry Banana Smoothie (Chapter 8), nettle tea with lemon and honey (optional)

Morning snack: 1 pint fresh berries

Lunch: 1 Veggie Burger (Chapter 10), chili from last night, large mixed-greens salad with your choice dressing (Chapter 11; optional)

Afternoon snack: 2 or 3 celery ribs

Dinner: Turkey Meatballs in Chunky Garden Vegetable Sauce (Chapter 13), cooked brown rice, baked sweet potato, large mixed-greens salad with your choice dressing (Chapter 11; optional)

Evening snack: 1 or 2 peaches

Day 3

Greet the day with a tall glass of water and a squeeze of lemon.

Breakfast: Easy Leftover Brown Rice Pudding (Chapter 9), Sunrise and Shine Juice (Chapter 7), dandelion tea with lemon and honey (optional)

Morning snack: 1 or 2 handfuls pumpkin seeds

Lunch: Tabbouleh Wraps (Chapter 10), baked sweet potato, large mixed-greens salad with your choice dressing (Chapter 11; optional)

Afternoon snack: 1 raw yellow bell pepper

Dinner: Hiziki Salad (Chapter 11), Asian Poached Chicken for One (Chapter 13), Old-Fashioned Scalloped Potatoes (Chapter 15)

Evening snack: 1 or 2 pears

Day 4

Greet the day with a tall glass of water and a squeeze of lemon.

Breakfast: Spelt Berry Porridge (Chapter 9), Bright-Eyed and Bushy-Tailed Juice (Chapter 7), fennel tea with lemon and honey (optional)

Morning snack: 1 handful Brazil nuts

Lunch: Italian-Style Three-Bean Salad (Chapter 11), Hippocrates Soup (Chapter 14), large mixed-greens salad with your choice dressing (Chapter 11; optional)

Afternoon snack: 1 pint cherry tomatoes

Dinner: Shepherd's Pie (Chapter 13), Red Radish Delight (Chapter 15), large mixed-greens salad with your choice dressing (Chapter 11; optional)

Evening snack: 1 or 2 apples

Day 5

Greet the day with a tall glass of water and a squeeze of lemon.

Breakfast: Breakfast Biscuits with Smoked Salmon (Chapter 9), Mineral-Rich Miso Soup (Chapter 14), Morning Refresher Juice (Chapter 7), sage tea with lemon and honey (optional)

Morning snack: 1 bunch grapes

Lunch: Minted Tomato Soup (Chapter 14); large mixed greens salad, fresh bean or seed sprouts, and your choice dressing (Chapter 11; optional)

Afternoon snack: 1 medium bowl of raw sauerkraut sprinkled with freshly ground flaxseeds

Dinner: Steamy Salmon Lasagna (Chapter 13), Crisp Nori Chips with Toasted Sesame Oil (Chapter 12), Roasted Vegetable Medley (Chapter 15), large mixed-greens salad with your choice dressing (Chapter 11; optional)

Evening snack: A few dates or plums

Day 6

Greet the day with a tall glass of water and a squeeze of lemon.

Breakfast: Perky Pumpkin Pancakes (Chapter 9), 1 pint fresh berries, Velvety Banana Smoothie (Chapter 8), nettle tea with lemon and honey (optional)

Morning snack: 1 pint cherry tomatoes

Lunch: White Bean Salad (Chapter 10), Tomato Soup with Lemon and Garlic (Chapter 14), Crisp Nori Chips with Toasted Sesame Oil (Chapter 12), celery and carrot sticks

Afternoon snack: 1 or more whole cucumbers

Dinner: Slow Cooker Cassoulet (Chapter 13), $\frac{1}{2}$ cup cooked brown rice, large mixed-greens salad with your choice dressing (Chapter 11; optional)

Evening snack: A few dates or plums

Day 7

Greet the day with a tall glass of water and a squeeze of lemon.

Breakfast: South-of-the-Border Breakfast Burritos (Chapter 9), Super Green Smoothie (Chapter 8), dandelion tea with lemon and honey (optional)

Morning snack: 1 wedge watermelon

Lunch: Leftover Slow Cooker Cassoulet (Chapter 13), Alkalizing Apple–Cucumber Salad (Chapter 11), Crisp Nori Chips with Toasted Sesame Oil (Chapter 12)

Afternoon snack: 2 or more whole carrots

Dinner: Slow-Cooked Red Lentil Curry (Chapter 13), $\frac{1}{2}$ cup cooked brown rice, large mixed-greens salad with your choice dressing (Chapter 11; optional)

Evening snack: A few dates or plums

Week 2

Congratulations on making it through your first week! You should be beginning to feel better already. Remember to substitute freely if you can't find something on the menu, and don't allow yourself to go hungry!

> **BALANCE BONUS**
>
> Feel free to play with the menus. Add a sprinkle of freshly ground flaxseed to salads and entrées, or top your oats or smoothies with chopped fruit or nuts.

Day 8

Greet the day with a tall glass of water and a squeeze of lemon.

Breakfast: Yummy Millet Mash (Chapter 15), Papaya Coconut Dream Smoothie (Chapter 8), fennel tea with lemon and honey (optional)

Morning snack: $\frac{1}{2}$ cantaloupe

Lunch: Vegetable Sushi Rolls (Chapter 15), leftover Slow-Cooked Red Lentil Curry (Chapter 13), pH-Style Tortilla Chips (Chapter 12), Wholly Guacamole (Chapter 12)

Afternoon snack: 1 pint fresh cherries and 1 handful almond slivers

Dinner: Vegetarian Butternut Squash Soup (Chapter 14), *Tarka Dhal* (Indian Spiced Lentils; Chapter 15), large mixed-greens salad with your choice dressing (Chapter 11; optional)

Evening snack: Wholly Guacamole (Chapter 12) with celery sticks

Day 9

Greet the day with a tall glass of water and a squeeze of lemon.

Breakfast: Quick Oats (Chapter 9) sprinkled with cinnamon and chopped walnuts, Morning Refresher Juice (Chapter 7), sage tea with lemon and honey (optional)

Morning snack: 2 or more carrots

Lunch: Greek Lentil and Fresh Dill Salad (Chapter 11), Tomato Soup with Lemon and Garlic (Chapter 14), pH-Style Tortilla Chips (Chapter 12), Wholly Guacamole (Chapter 12)

Afternoon snack: 1 apple and 2 celery ribs

Dinner: Spicy Thai Soup with Coconut Milk (Chapter 14), Asian Tempeh Cutlet Salad (Chapter 13), large mixed-greens salad with your choice dressing (Chapter 11; optional)

Evening snack: 1 handful almonds

Day 10

Greet the day with a tall glass of water and a squeeze of lemon.

Breakfast: Savory Quinoa Breakfast Bowl (Chapter 9), Revved-Up Reviving Juice (Chapter 7), nettle tea with lemon and honey (optional)

Morning snack: 1 pint blueberries

Lunch: Jamaican Bean and Veggie Salad (Chapter 11), Roasted Vegetable Medley (Chapter 15), leftover Spicy Thai Soup with Coconut Milk (Chapter 14)

Afternoon snack: Fresh pineapple spears

Dinner: Cream of Carrot Soup (Chapter 14), Whitefish with Braised Fennel (Chapter 13), large mixed-greens salad with your choice dressing (Chapter 11; optional)

Evening snack: 1 or 2 fresh pears

Day 11

Greet the day with a tall glass of water and a squeeze of lemon.

Breakfast: Spelt Berry Porridge (Chapter 9), Coconut Caribbean Cream Smoothie (Chapter 8), dandelion tea with lemon and honey (optional)

Morning snack: $\frac{1}{2}$ cantaloupe

Lunch: Leafy Tuna Lunch (Chapter 10), leftover Cream of Carrot Soup (Chapter 14), red bell pepper rings

Afternoon snack: 1 ripe mango

Dinner: Simply Salmon for One (Chapter 13), leftover cooked brown rice, large mixed-greens salad with your choice dressing (Chapter 11; optional)

Evening snack: Cut raw vegetables with Garlicky Cucumber Dip (Chapter 12)

Day 12

Greet the day with a tall glass of water and a squeeze of lemon.

Breakfast: Easy Leftover Brown Rice Pudding (Chapter 9), Piña Colada Smoothie (Chapter 8), nettle tea with lemon and honey (optional)

Morning snack: Cucumber spears and carrot sticks

Lunch: Beet Salad with Sweet Potato (Chapter 10), Hippocrates Soup (Chapter 14), Spiced Roasted Nut Mix (Chapter 12)

Afternoon snack: 1 ripe avocado

Dinner: 1 Lemony Chicken Burger (Chapter 13), large mixed-greens salad with your choice dressing (Chapter 11; optional)

Evening snack: Cut raw vegetables with Hearty Spinach Dip (Chapter 12)

Day 13

Greet the day with a tall glass of water and a squeeze of lemon.

Breakfast: Breakfast Biscuits with Smoked Salmon (Chapter 9), Citrus Circus Juice (Chapter 7), fennel tea with lemon and honey (optional)

Morning snack: 1 handful almonds

Lunch: Quick Quinoa Bowl (Chapter 10), Dashi (Chapter 14), Crisp Nori Chips with Toasted Sesame Oil (Chapter 12)

Afternoon snack: 1 pint cherry tomatoes

Dinner: Zippy Lentil Soup (Chapter 14), Zucchini and Quinoa with Chickpea Sauce (Chapter 15), large mixed-greens salad with your choice dressing (Chapter 11; optional)

Evening snack: Very Veggie Smoothie (Chapter 8)

Day 14

Greet the day with a tall glass of water and a squeeze of lemon.

Breakfast: Perky Pumpkin Pancakes (Chapter 9), Green Machine Juice (Chapter 7), sage tea with lemon and honey (optional)

Morning snack: 1 bunch grapes

Lunch: Tuna Steak with Kale and Caper Dressing (Chapter 10), Minted Tomato Soup (Chapter 14), Spiced Roasted Nut Mix (Chapter 12)

Afternoon snack: 1 or 2 apples

Dinner: Potato and Leek Soup (Chapter 14), large mixed-greens salad with your choice dressing (Chapter 11; optional)

Evening snack: Cut raw vegetables with Baba Ghanoush (Chapter 12)

Week 3

Congratulations! You've made it through 2 weeks and should be seeing and feeling some amazing results. If your pH is testing well and you're still not feeling the improvement you'd hoped for, you might need to adjust your menu.

Rashes, headaches, fluid retention, an inability to lose weight, "brain fog," or chronic stomach upsets are often a result of a hidden food allergy. The most common food allergens are cow's milk dairy products, eggs, chocolate, strawberries, wheat, soy and peanut products, and nightshades—potatoes, tomatoes, sweet and hot peppers, eggplant, tomatillos, tamarillos, pepinos, pimentos, paprika, and tobacco.

The menus in this book contain few, if any, of these foods, with the exception of the nightshade plants and soy products. So if you're still experiencing nagging problems, try eliminating soy products and nightshades for at least the next 2 weeks. In the case of nightshade allergies, eliminate the foods for an extended period—even a month or more—to see significant improvement.

ACID ALERT!

If you cut out questionable food allergens and your condition improves, *do not reintroduce them without first consulting with a physician.* Allergens can provoke a rapidly progressing allergic reaction, which can lead to anaphylactic shock and even death.

Each day of week 3, continue to plan for your meals. Keep up with your journal, noting any changes in how you feel. Make time to get a little fresh air and exercise, and be sure to get enough rest. Stay hydrated, too.

Suggested menus for this week progressively become lighter and more alkalizing than previous menus. You may find this change brings rapid improvement to your sense of well-being, or it may feel too drastic. Stay within your comfort zone so you don't give up and go completely off target.

Day 15

Greet the day with a tall glass of water and a squeeze of lemon.

Breakfast: Quick Oats (Chapter 9) sprinkled with cinnamon, raisins, and chopped walnuts; Ruby Rush Juice (Chapter 7); dandelion tea with lemon and honey (optional)

Morning snack: 1 or 2 apples

Lunch: Leftover Potato and Leek Soup (Chapter 14), large mixed-greens salad with your choice dressing (Chapter 11; optional)

Afternoon snack: 1 handful mixed nuts

Dinner: pH Pizza Pockets (Chapter 12), Italian Fish Stew (Chapter 14), large mixed-greens salad with your choice dressing (Chapter 11; optional)

Evening snack: Cut raw vegetables with Baba Ghanoush (Chapter 12)

Day 16

Greet the day with a tall glass of water and a squeeze of lemon.

Breakfast: Blend until smooth: 1 pint fresh washed berries, 1 banana, and 1 tablespoon ground flaxseed; Quick Oats (Chapter 9), if still hungry; organic herbal tea

Morning snack: 1 large fresh vegetable juice of choice

Lunch: Tabbouleh Wraps (Chapter 10), Mineral-Rich Miso Soup (Chapter 14), large mixed-greens salad with your choice dressing (Chapter 11; optional)

Afternoon snack: 1 large fresh vegetable juice of choice

Dinner: Curried Chickpea and Spinach Stew (Chapter 14), large mixed-greens salad with your choice dressing (Chapter 11; optional)

Evening snack: Cut raw vegetables with Wholly Guacamole (Chapter 12)

Day 17

Greet the day with a tall glass of water and a squeeze of lemon.

Breakfast: Juice together: 1 celery rib, 1 cucumber, and 1 carrot; 1 pint blueberries; organic herbal tea

Morning snack: 1 large fresh vegetable juice of choice

Lunch: Leftover Curried Chickpea and Spinach Stew (Chapter 14), large mixed-greens salad with your choice dressing (Chapter 11; optional)

Afternoon snack: 1 large fresh vegetable juice of choice

Dinner: Slow Cooker Cassoulet (Chapter 13), large mixed-greens salad with your choice dressing (Chapter 11; optional)

Evening snack: pH-Style Tortilla Chips (Chapter 12) with Wholly Guacamole (Chapter 12)

Day 18

Greet the day with a tall glass of water and a squeeze of lemon.

Breakfast: Juice together 4 celery ribs, 1 cucumber, and $\frac{1}{2}$ apple, and stir in 1 teaspoon green vegetable powder; $\frac{1}{2}$ cantaloupe; organic herbal tea

Morning snack: 1 large fresh vegetable juice of choice

Lunch: Leftover Slow Cooker Cassoulet (Chapter 13), large mixed-greens salad with your choice dressing (Chapter 11; optional)

Afternoon snack: 1 large fresh vegetable juice of choice

Dinner: Slow-Cooked Red Lentil Curry (Chapter 13), large mixed-greens salad with your choice dressing (Chapter 11; optional)

Evening snack: Crisp Nori Chips with Toasted Sesame Oil (Chapter 12)

Day 19

Greet the day with a tall glass of water and a squeeze of lemon.

Breakfast: Green Goddess Juice (Chapter 7), Quick Oats (Chapter 9), organic herbal tea

Morning snack: 1 large fresh vegetable juice of choice

Lunch: Tabbouleh Wraps (Chapter 10), Mineral-Rich Miso Soup (Chapter 14), large mixed-greens salad with your choice dressing (Chapter 11; optional)

Afternoon snack: 1 large fresh vegetable juice of choice

Dinner: Curried Chickpea and Spinach Stew (Chapter 14), large mixed-greens salad with your choice dressing (Chapter 11; optional)

Evening snack: Crisp Nori Chips with Toasted Sesame Oil (Chapter 12)

Day 20

Greet the day with a tall glass of water and a squeeze of lemon.

Breakfast: Green Goddess Juice (Chapter 7), Quick Oats (Chapter 9), organic herbal tea

Morning snack: 1 large fresh vegetable juice

Lunch: Jamaican Bean and Veggie Salad (Chapter 11), cut raw vegetables, Wholly Guacamole (Chapter 12)

Afternoon snack: 1 large fresh vegetable juice

Dinner: Spicy Thai Soup with Coconut Milk (Chapter 14), large mixed-greens salad with your choice dressing (Chapter 11; optional)

Evening snack: Crisp Nori Chips with Toasted Sesame Oil (Chapter 12)

Day 21

Greet the day with a tall glass of water and a squeeze of lemon.

Breakfast: Good-Morning Grapefruit Smoothie (Chapter 8), Quick Oats (Chapter 9), organic herbal tea

Morning snack: 1 large fresh vegetable juice of choice

Lunch: Leftover Spicy Thai Soup with Coconut Milk (Chapter 14), cut raw vegetables, Garlicky Cucumber Dip (Chapter 12)

Afternoon snack: 1 large fresh vegetable juice of choice

Dinner: Asian Tempeh Cutlet Salad (Chapter 13), Onion Wakame Casserole (Chapter 15), large mixed-greens salad with your choice dressing (Chapter 11; optional)

Evening snack: Crisp Nori Chips with Toasted Sesame Oil (Chapter 12)

Week 4

Weeks 1 and 2 are meant to be a gentle introduction to the pH balance way of eating, week 3 helps you delve deeper into its benefits, and week 4 is a special bonus. Use this week either as a personal "pH retreat" or as an emergency correction if you find you've gone too far off track. By the end of this week, you'll undoubtedly feel like a brand-new you!

BALANCE BONUS

To improve your results during week 4, add dry skin brushing, an alkalizing bath, light exercise, deep breathing, and meditation to your regimen. You also may want to include extra lemon water, 32 ounces fresh vegetable juice, and green vegetable drink powder. You don't have to add these all at once, but the more you include, the better you'll feel.

Day 1

If you're reading through week 4 because you need to get back on track, it's likely you had trouble balancing the time required to prepare your meals. This week is much easier. Your cooking and planning skills will improve over time, but for now, follow the guidelines for this week, and you'll be balancing once again.

Begin every day with a large glass of water and a squeeze of fresh lemon, followed by a warm herbal tea. Then pack two packets of instant miso soup to take with you if you're going to work.

If you find that food preparation has been cumbersome, make a trip to the grocery store and buy a prepared platter of cut vegetables and a large premade fruit salad bowl. The fruit will be your breakfast. The vegetables are for snacking and lunch.

At lunchtime, heat some water and make your miso soup. Enjoy it with your fresh vegetables.

After work, get a little exercise. Go for a 20-minute walk or crank up your favorite music and dance. Move, breathe, laugh, and sing out loud.

Make a huge salad for dinner using a prewashed bag of baby greens and your leftover cut vegetables. Top it with a squeeze of fresh lemon and any seeds, sprouts, or nuts you have around. Accompany it by a glass of fresh juice made with 1 cucumber, 2 ribs celery, 4 carrots, 1 apple, and 1 ($\frac{1}{2}$-inch) piece fresh ginger. After dinner, relax a bit with some quiet reading or music. Take an alkalizing bath and tuck into bed by 10 P.M.

Days 2 Through 7

You could follow the instructions for day 1 for the rest of the week, but that would be boring. You'd be missing out on nutritional variety, too. Instead, begin each day with some warm lemon water, followed by your choice of herbal tea. Have a couple grapefruit for breakfast, or your choice of purchased or homemade fruit salads. If you're extra hungry, wait a few minutes and have a bowl of oatmeal, too.

For a morning snack break, pack a couple whole fruits, like apples, pears, or bananas. Also make a large vegetable juice to take along. If you really dislike juicing, you can buy premade vegetable juices, as long as they're organic and contain no added sugar.

For lunch and afternoon snacking, pack or buy some leafy salad greens and crunchy veggies. Also pack along your miso soup packets or a premade, no-additive organic vegetarian soup.

After work, exercise for 20 to 30 minutes. Consider rebounding, which is easy on the joints and is excellent at stimulating lymph circulation. Walking or cycling in the fresh air also are great.

After exercise, make a huge glass of your favorite vegetable juice, and enjoy it with a simple supper of roasted mixed vegetables, slow-cooked beans or grains, and a large fresh salad. After dinner, relax, take an alkalizing bath, and be in bed by 10 P.M.

The Least You Need to Know

- If you follow a pH balance diet and don't feel improvement, you might be suffering from a hidden food allergy. Try eliminating soy foods and nightshades to see if these may be the culprits.
- Add alkalizing activities and supplements to your regimen to get the most out of your pH dieting experience.
- Plan your days and your meals to keep them as simple as possible to reap the greatest benefits and to assure your diet stays on track.

Shopping and Kitchen Savvy

In This Chapter

- Helpful shopping hints
- Storing your bounty
- Cooking with dried beans and grains
- Prepping for success

Not long ago (my grandmother's generation, to be precise), if you wanted to cook something, you had to start from scratch. Premade foods and mixes weren't around then. If you wanted to eat spaghetti, for example, you (or someone nearby) had to make the pasta. If you wanted to eat a sandwich, you (or someone nearby) had to bake the bread. If you wanted mayonnaise on your sandwich, you (or someone) had to make that, too. Cooking then was much more labor intensive than it is now. But Grandma had lots of tricks up her sleeve!

What my grandmother knew that few people of this generation know was how to shop smartly, how to prepare some foods ahead of time in order to make meals come together more easily, and how to preserve and store food for when either her time or fresh foods would be in short supply. Because a pH balance diet does not allow for much in the way of prepackaged foods, Grandma's tricks will come in handy. This chapter will explore the many tried-and-true techniques that will make your dieting experience a doable and pleasant adventure.

Smart Shopping

Almost all the food in a pH balance diet is easy to find at your local supermarket or farmers' market. A few unusual items may be a little more difficult to find, such as specialty grains, flours, or oils. These are usually best found in your local health food store. If you don't have a health food store near you, all is not lost. Even difficult-to-locate items can be found readily online, and Appendix B lists such online sources.

Beyond that, I encourage you to check around your area for a *CSA* (community-supported agriculture) group. CSAs provide an easy method of obtaining regular deliveries of the freshest local, seasonal food available. CSA shares are usually competitively priced because the arrangement removes several layers of middlemen. Many CSA farmers also provide organic eggs, fish, and poultry.

DEFINITION

In **CSA** (community-supported agriculture), a farmer sells a certain number of "shares" to the public. In exchange for purchasing a membership in the CSA, members receive a box (or a bag or basket) of seasonal produce each week throughout the farming season. Shares normally consist of vegetables, but other farm products may be included as well. To find a CSA near you, visit localharvest.org.

When purchasing meat, try to locate a true local source. Is there a slaughterhouse nearby that services local ranchers? That is an excellent place to begin your search for meat that has been carefully raised and recently butchered. If you live near a fishing community, take a trip to the docks one day and purchase your seafood directly from the fisherman—you will never find anything so fresh in a grocery store cooler!

There are a few key guidelines to follow when shopping for fresh produce. Produce should be purchased once a week, at a minimum. For most people, shopping more often than that is a burden. But if you can manage to shop for your fresh fruits and vegetables once per week, and not buy more than you are able to consume, you can keep yourself well supplied with high-quality produce that has not gone past its prime.

Try to buy your produce from local growers when it is in season. Buying local, seasonal produce ensures that your produce is of high quality, and it has not been picked before it was ripe so that it could be shipped to you from the other side of the planet. It will cost less and be a better nutritional value, too.

If you're buying produce in a grocery store, watch the prices. Often the best sales coincide with what is in season and locally grown. Get to know the produce manager. This person can answer lots of questions and place orders for your special requests. Lastly, learn to read the stickers. Those little stickers on your fruit and vegetables always state variety and origin. Are your grapes organically raised in California? Or were they heavily sprayed in the fields of Chile? Opt for organic produce when you can.

When fresh fruits and vegetables are not available, choose frozen over canned goods, and organic over nonorganic. Remember to read ingredient labels to avoid added sugar, salt, dyes, artificial flavorings, and preservatives.

And of course, if you have the time and the space, by all means experiment with growing your own food. The food that you raise and care for is food that you know you can depend on to be life-giving, fresh, and chemical free. As a bonus, the modest exercise you get from gardening will help to balance your pH, too.

Storing and Preparing Fresh Produce

As soon as you get home with your fresh produce, get straight to work on putting it away. Properly prepared and stored fruits and vegetables last longer and make meal preparations a breeze.

Here are some tips on storing and prepping fresh produce:

Root vegetables (beets, carrots, ginger, radishes, turnips): Place in your refrigerator's crisper drawer, loosely wrapped in a plastic produce bag.

Peppers (bell and chile): Store whole, in the crisper drawer. Eat, cook, or freeze within a few days.

Celery, fennel, and rhubarb: Remove from plastic produce bags, lay on a length of aluminum foil, roll foil tightly around the stalks, crimp the ends shut, and store in the crisper drawer. When you're ready to use, take out just what you need and rewrap the rest.

Leafy greens: Separate leaves and swish around, submerged, in a sink full of water. Lift out into a bowl, clean out any sand or grit from the sink, and repeat until no grit remains. Drain well, wrap in paper towels, and store in a plastic bag in the refrigerator for up to 3 or 4 days.

Leeks: Leave in the plastic produce bag and place in the crisper drawer. When ready to use, trim off and discard the roots and tough green leaf ends, split the leek lengthwise, and rinse like other leafy greens. Cut leaves to desired thickness and cook immediately.

Onions and garlic: Hang in mesh bags in a cool, dark place. If you buy loose onions and garlic, store them in the same manner in a clean pair of women's stockings.

Potatoes: These can be refrigerated, but red (new) potatoes eventually become waxy, and white potatoes may develop a grainy texture. Both types will acquire sweet taste over time if refrigerated. Ideally, store in a mesh or paper sack in a cool, dark place away from onions.

Tomatoes: Store upside down on a counter or on the windowsill if they're not yet ripe.

 ACID ALERT!

Greens lose their nutrients rapidly and are best consumed or cooked immediately. And never refrigerate tomatoes. They'll become pithy and flavorless.

Fruit (most): Refrigerate fruit, but don't wash it until you're ready to use it. Keep citrus fruits in produce bags to keep them from drying out.

As you are working with your produce, be sure to take a little time to trim some radishes, slice some bell pepper rings, and make a batch of carrot and celery sticks. Store them in separate zipper-lock plastic bags or other plastic containers. This will save you some prep time later and ensure you always have ready-cut salad fixings and snacks for taking to work.

Also store a quantity of diced onion, bell pepper, and celery in zipper-lock plastic bags in the freezer. These are staple seasoning vegetables in many cuisines, and it's nice to be able to pull them out of the freezer, already chopped, when you're ready to cook!

Dried Goods, Beans, and Grains

You will not consume much flour on an alkalizing diet, and the flour that you will use will not be modern wheat flour—not even whole-grain wheat flour—because such flour is very acid forming. Some of the flours that are allowed in moderation include kamut, spelt, and chickpea flour. These flours are most readily available at health food stores and online. Whatever you do, do not overbuy flours. They rapidly lose their nutritional value after they have been ground and may even go rancid. Buy your flours in small amounts, allowing for a little experimentation with recipes, and you will not end up losing money on flour that is no longer good to use. Alternatively, you can mill flours from whole grains yourself, as you need them.

Dried beans, on the other hand, are something that you can buy in bulk if you have room to store them. The same goes for whole grains. Dried beans keep well over long periods of time, and they will save you quite a bit of money over the canned and frozen varieties. Store your beans and grains in a cool, dry place, either in their original bags or in glass jars.

Dried beans and legumes are easy to cook, but like everything else, you have to know what you're doing. There are three methods for cooking dried beans:

Overnight soak: Rinse and sort the beans to get rid of any stones and debris. Place the beans in a large pot, cover with cold water, and allow them to sit overnight. The next day, drain the beans, and using fresh water, proceed with your recipe.

Fast soak: Rinse and sort beans. Place beans in a large pot, cover with cold water, and bring to a boil over high heat. Boil for 2 minutes, cover, and remove from heat. Allow the beans to sit for 2 hours. Drain, and using fresh water, proceed with your recipe.

In the slow cooker: Rinse and sort 1 pound of beans. Place in a slow cooker, add 6 cups water and seasonings, if desired. Cover, set to high, and cook for 5 or 6 hours.

ACID ALERT!

Regardless of which method you choose, wait until the beans are tender before adding any acidic recipe ingredients—vinegars, in particular. Beans that come into contact with acids before they have cooked through may never become tender.

The slow cooker method is my favorite because I can create a meal for a crowd with nearly no effort whatsoever. Plus, I can cook a pound of beans without any seasoning and store them in the refrigerator for use in other recipes, such as soups and salads.

I always try to keep a stash of slow-cooked beans in a zipper-lock plastic bag in my refrigerator. They are handy for creating any number of healthy alkalizing meals, and they will greatly reduce the amount of time you spend in meal preparation. Because I've cooked them from scratch, I also enjoy knowing they contain no added salt or unhealthy fats and preservatives.

Rice and other grains are also good to make ahead and store in the refrigerator or freezer. The easiest method for cooking rice is to use an electric rice cooker. But this method doesn't always work well with brown rice because it needs to steam for a longer time than white rice. And when you're trying to balance pH, brown rice is, by far, preferred over white. Using a pressure cooker instead saves you time and ensures fully cooked rice, too.

To cook brown rice in a pressure cooker, rinse and sort rice, and place 2 parts rice in the pressure cooker, along with 3 parts cold water. Add a postage stamp–size piece of kombu, and stir once. Add the lid, lock, and bring to pressure over high heat. Reduce the temperature to low, and cook for 45 minutes. Allow the pressure to come down naturally before opening the lid.

Other grains come with instructions for their particular methods of preparation printed on their containers. Be sure to reference these because each is a little different.

ACID ALERT!

When preparing quinoa, rinse it several times before cooking. Quinoa is coated with a powdery, bitter-tasting saponin resin that must be washed away before cooking.

pH-Friendly Cooking Methods

Everyone has heard that people should avoid fried foods and opt for broiled, steamed, or braised food instead. But not everyone realizes how much cooking methods alone can affect a meal's nutritional value.

Slow cooker cooking is an excellent carefree and gentle way of preparing meals. Because of the low slow-cooking temperatures, many of the food's vitamins are retained that would otherwise be destroyed.

Stir-frying is another good way to quickly cook meats, seafood, and vegetables. Although the temperatures are high, little oil is used, and the foods are quickly finished to a just-cooked, tender-crisp state. Stir-frying retains much of a food's vitamin content, as well as meat's protein integrity. When using the stir-fry method of cooking, always use a stable oil like virgin coconut oil.

Water sautéing enables you to have the flavor of sautéed vegetables without using heated oils. Exposing polyunsaturated vegetable oils to high heat can result in the production of oxidized compounds and free radicals detrimental to your health.

Healthy food expert George Mateljan is an advocate of water-sautéing foods. He advocates adding healthy oils to foods after they have been cooked, which not only maintains the health-promoting nutrients in the oil, but also increases the satiation factor and flavor of foods.

To water sauté vegetables, heat the recommended amount of water or broth (using the recommended oil amount as a guide) in a stainless-steel skillet over medium heat. When the water begins to steam, add the vegetables, cover, and cook for the recommended time—usually from 3 to 5 minutes. If you want to eliminate excess liquid, cook uncovered for a few more minutes. Remove from heat, and toss vegetables with extra-virgin olive oil or coconut oil.

The Least You Need to Know

- Learning to shop smartly, prepare some foods ahead of time, and store food for when your time or fresh foods will be limited are all great ways to keep your diet on track.
- Shop regularly, join a CSA, and even try growing some of your own produce to ensure your success on the pH balance diet.
- Slow cookers and pressure cookers can save you tons of time and effort.

pH Balance
Recipes

The thought of pH balance recipes might bring to mind lab coats and Bunsen burners, but balancing the pH of your diet doesn't require any scientific background.

The recipes in Part 3 include everything from breakfasts worth waking up for to desserts you'll crave and everything in between: lunches, salads, soups and stews, dinners, sides, and snacks—even nourishing juices and sensational smoothies. I give you 101 recipes to help you easily—and deliciously—adapt and thrive on a pH balance diet.

Nourishing Juices

In This Chapter

- The advantages of juicing
- Fitting in fruits and vegetables
- Super-juicing basics
- Juice recipes for fun, health, and variety

According to the U.S. Department of Agriculture, you should consume between three and five servings of vegetables and two to four servings of fruit every day—at a minimum, which isn't always easy. That's where juicing comes in. Juicing provides a simple way to fulfill your daily fruit and vegetable requirements, in an easily absorbed, life-enhancing form. Regularly drinking fresh fruit and vegetable juice can help increase your vitality, boost your energy levels, and help your body fight disease.

Sure, you could just eat a salad or have an apple every day instead. But juicing allows you to consume far more nutrition-packed fresh produce than you could ever consume whole. Imagine all the chewing involved in consuming $\frac{1}{2}$ pound of raw carrots—not to mention how full you'd feel! You can easily drink that same $\frac{1}{2}$ pound of carrots in juice form. Plus, a juicer is more efficient at breaking open a vegetable's cell walls than your teeth are able to do. Juicing makes every drop of nutrition instantly available to you.

What's more, when you juice fresh fruit and vegetables and drink their juicy goodness immediately, you get a bigger nutritional bang for your buck, especially compared to commercially prepared store-bought juices that have been heat-treated (pasteurized) and stripped of their vital enzymes. Fresh juice contains no artificial additives and preservatives, and you can mix and match ingredients as you like.

No single food can provide all the nutrition you need to stay healthy, so juicing and drinking a wide variety of fruits and vegetables enables you to get all the alkalizing nutrients your body needs, in all the flavor varieties and nutrient combinations you can imagine.

The easiest way to start juicing is to use the fruits and vegetables you like to eat. If it's summertime and you have loads of garden-fresh cucumbers on hand, for example, make cucumber juice. If you find that's a little bland, add a bit of lemon juice to liven it up. With a little experimentation, you'll soon have a few juice recipes you enjoy.

Juicing Tips from the Pros

Dr. Ann Wigmore, the mother of the raw-foods movement, taught that there's no approach to dieting that's more naturally alkalizing than eating raw fruits and vegetables—especially leafy greens.

Dr. Wigmore recommended including a variety of chlorophyll-rich, green sprouted seeds, grasses, and other leafy vegetables in her juices. On their own, or as additions to other juices, each of these provide phenomenal health benefits:

- Wheatgrass (extremely sweet)
- Barley grass (slightly bitter)
- Sprouts: alfalfa, sunflower seed, mung bean, etc.
- Leafy greens: kale, spinach, romaine lettuce, etc.

Another juicing expert was Dr. Max Gerson. His amazing juice therapy has been shown to miraculously cure cases of illness and disease that had been abandoned by mainstream medical doctors. He recommended drinking one 6- to 8-ounce glass of freshly squeezed juice hourly, each day, as follows:

- First juice of the day: Freshly squeezed orange juice
- Juices 2, 6, 8, and 12: Green juice made with any combination of romaine lettuce, chard, young beet tops, watercress, red cabbage, endive, escarole; ¼ small green pepper; and 1 medium apple
- Juices 3, 4, 7, 11, and 13: Apple/carrot juice made with equal amounts of each
- Juices 5, 9, and 10: Plain carrot juice

Both Dr. Gerson's and Dr. Wigmore's philosophies on nutrition and healing foods have proven highly successful, but they're just the beginning of the exciting adventure juicing can be. Try out the delicious energizing recipes in this chapter, and have fun experimenting!

Sunrise and Shine Juice

This juice, brimming with tropical-flavored nutrition, is packed with alkalizing potassium, vitamin C, and other heart-healthy and cancer-fighting antioxidants!

Yield:	Prep time:	Serving size:	
about 2 cups	5 minutes	about 1 cup	
Each serving has:			
41.4g carbohydrate	0.4g fat	4.6g fiber	1g protein

1 medium ripe mango, peeled and seeded	1 medium orange, peeled
	½ medium pomegranate, peeled

1. Cut mango and orange into pieces that will fit into your juicer's feed tube.

2. Juice mango and orange together, and pour into glasses.

3. Reserving 1 tablespoon pomegranate seeds, juice remainder of pomegranate, and pour into orange-mango juice. Juices will separate to give a pretty sunrise effect.

4. Garnish with reserved pomegranate seeds, and serve at room temperature or chilled.

Bright-Eyed and Bushy-Tailed Juice

This pleasant, mild-flavored juice is full of carotenoids that support eye and skin health.

Yield:	Prep time:	Cook time:	Serving size:
about 2 cups	5 minutes	10 minutes	about 1 cup

Each serving has:			
15.5g carbohydrate	0.2g fat	3g fiber	0.5g protein

1 bag green tea	1 medium apple, washed
½ cup boiling water	Handful fresh parsley
1 medium carrot, washed and trimmed	

1. Place green tea bag in boiling water, cover, and allow to steep for 10 minutes.

2. Remove and discard tea bag, and allow green tea to cool for a few minutes.

3. Cut carrot and apple into pieces that will fit into your juicer's feed tube.

4. Ball up parsley, and push it through your juicer's feed tube using apple and carrot pieces.

5. Stir juice into green tea, pour into glasses, and serve warm or chilled.

BALANCE BONUS

Save the pulp left over from juicing fruits and vegetables in a zipper-lock plastic bag in your refrigerator or freezer. The pulp is full of healthy, natural fiber you can add to meatloaves, breads, stews, and other dishes to boost your nutrient intake and support colon health.

Morning Refresher Juice

Cool, cleansing apple, melon, and kiwi dominate the fresh flavors of this good-start juice.

Yield:	Prep time:	Serving size:	
about 2 cups	5 minutes	about 1 cup	
Each serving has:			
41.5g carbohydrate	0.8g fat	5g fiber	2.1g protein

½ medium peach, pitted

1 small apple, washed

¼ medium honeydew melon, peeled

½ medium kiwi, skin on

1 handful green grapes, washed

1. Cut peach, apple, and honeydew melon into pieces that will fit into your juicer's feed tube.

2. Juice peach, apple, honeydew melon, kiwi, and green grapes together.

3. Pour into glasses, and serve at room temperature or chilled.

PHABULOUS PHACT

This juice is both cleansing and diuretic. Melon helps clear the skin while it flushes the kidneys, bladder, and intestines. Plus, grape skins contain toning tannins that stimulate a healthy appetite.

Revved-Up Reviving Juice

The bright kick of ginger will wake up your system and stimulate your circulation.

Yield:	Prep time:	Serving size:
about 2 cups	5 minutes	about 1 cup

Each serving has:			
20.4g carbohydrate	0.3g fat	4.5g fiber	1.5g protein

2 small beets, washed and trimmed

1 medium carrot, washed and trimmed

1 medium pear

½ medium lime, peeled if not organic

1 (1-in.) piece fresh ginger

1. Cut beets, carrot, and pear into pieces that will fit into your juicer's feed tube.

2. Juice beets, carrot, pear, lime, and ginger together.

3. Pour into glasses, and serve at room temperature or chilled.

PHABULOUS PHACT

Beets have a high potassium content, which is both alkalizing and helpful in lowering high blood pressure.

Citrus Circus Juice

Enjoy the riotous blend of citrus flavors in this celebration of vitamin C.

Yield:	Prep time:	Serving size:	
about 2 cups	5 minutes	about 1 cup	
Each serving has:			
16g carbohydrate	0.2g fat	2.9g fiber	1.3g protein

1 medium pink or red grapefruit, peeled

1 medium orange, peeled

½ medium lemon, peeled if not organic

½ medium lime, peeled if not organic

1. Cut grapefruit and orange into pieces that will fit into your juicer's feed tube.

2. Juice grapefruit, orange, lemon, and lime together.

3. Pour into glasses, and serve at room temperature or chilled.

PHABULOUS PHACT

Vitamin C helps bond iron to hemoglobin in red blood cells and assists in the absorption of calcium, helping you say good-bye to anemia and osteoporosis!

Ruby Rush Juice

Wake up to a rosy, berry-flavored citrus punch with this antioxidant-packed juice.

Yield:	Prep time:	Serving size:	
about 2 cups	5 minutes	about 1 cup	
Each serving has:			
12.5g carbohydrate	0.5g fat	4.7g fiber	1.1g protein

1 medium ruby red grapefruit, peeled	1 cup fresh raspberries, rinsed
	1 cup fresh cranberries, rinsed

1. Cut ruby red grapefruit into pieces that will fit into your juicer's feed tube.

2. Juice ruby red grapefruit, raspberries, and cranberries together.

3. Pour into glasses, and serve at room temperature or chilled.

> **BALANCE BONUS**
>
> When juicing citrus fruits, be sure to leave the white pith on the fruit. Citrus pith is full of healthy bioflavonoids that help with the absorption of vitamin C.

Summertime Cooler Juice

Cucumber is a refreshing green vegetable famous for its flavorful cooling properties in the cuisines of hot, humid tropical cultures.

Yield:	Prep time:	Serving size:	
about 2 cups	5 minutes	about 1 cup	
Each serving has:			
27.9g carbohydrate	0.4g fat	4.8g fiber	1g protein

½ medium cucumber, washed, and peeled if not organic

2 medium green apples, washed

1 small handful fresh cilantro

1. Cut cucumber and green apples into pieces that will fit into your juicer's feed tube.

2. Ball up cilantro, and push it through your juicer's feed tube using cucumber and apple pieces.

3. Pour into glasses, and serve at room temperature or chilled.

ACID ALERT!

Take care in selecting your produce. Opt for organic when possible. Several fruits and vegetables are so routinely contaminated with excessive amounts of pesticides and other harmful chemicals they've come to be known as the "dirty dozen": apples, bell peppers, carrots, celery, cherries, grapes (imported, especially Chilean), kale, lettuce, nectarines, peaches, pears, and strawberries. Choose organic of these foods especially.

Green Machine Juice

The garden-fresh flavors of these cleansing greens burst through to provide a quick energy boost for a midday snack.

Yield:	Prep time:	Serving size:	
about 1½ cups	2 minutes	about ¾ cup	
Each serving has:			
29.5g carbohydrate	0.6g fat	6.1g fiber	2g protein

1 medium zucchini, washed

2 medium apples, washed

1 generous handful baby spinach leaves

1 generous handful fresh alfalfa sprouts

1 large celery rib, washed

1. Cut zucchini and apples into pieces that will fit into your juicer's feed tube.

2. Ball up baby spinach leaves and alfalfa sprouts, and push them through your juicer's feed tube using zucchini, apple, and celery rib pieces.

3. Pour into glasses, and serve at room temperature or chilled.

PHABULOUS PHACT

Healthful, alkalizing spinach contains about twice as much iron as other greens and is a rich source of beta-carotene, vitamin E, the B-complex vitamins, vitamin C, calcium, magnesium, potassium, zinc, and iodine. It's also an excellent source of the blood purifier chlorophyll. No wonder Popeye was so healthy and strong!

Green Goddess Juice

The light, minty freshness of this super juice belies the many serious benefits it provides.

Yield:	Prep time:	Serving size:	
about 2 cups	5 minutes	about 1 cup	
Each serving has:			
16.8g carbohydrate	0.4g fat	1.9g fiber	1.9g protein

1 generous handful baby spinach leaves

2 large sprigs fresh mint

Several sprigs fresh parsley

½ medium *Galia melon*

1. Cut melon into pieces that will fit into your juicer's feed tube.

2. Ball up baby spinach leaves, mint, and parsley, and push them through your juicer's feed tube using Galia melon pieces.

3. Pour into glasses, and serve at room temperature or chilled.

Variation: If you can't find Galia melon, you can substitute the same amount of honeydew or cantaloupe instead.

DEFINITION

Galia melon is the first hybrid melon created from intensely fragrant Middle Eastern melons. Galias look like cantaloupe on the outside and honeydew on the inside. The flesh is smooth, light green, and sweet.

Tummy Tamer Juice

Lively ginger and pineapple provide tasty natural relief for slight stomach upsets or nausea.

Yield:	Prep time:	Serving size:	
about 2 cups	5 minutes	about 1 cup	
Each serving has:			
33.2g carbohydrate	0.5g fat	3.7g fiber	1.6g protein

½ medium pineapple, leaves removed and peeled, but not cored

¼ medium lemon, peeled if not organic

1 (1-in.) piece fresh ginger

1. Cut pineapple into long wedges that will fit into your juicer's feed tube.

2. Juice pineapple, lemon, and ginger together.

3. Pour into glasses, and serve at room temperature or chilled.

PHABULOUS PHACT

Ginger is a medicinal herb that possesses anti-inflammatory properties and helps reduce the pain of osteo- and rheumatoid arthritis. It also aids in colon cleansing, reduces spasms and cramping, and improves circulation. If that wasn't enough, this antioxidant, antimicrobial herb can even break fevers and relieve headaches, hot flashes, morning sickness, indigestion, nausea, and vomiting.

Super Smoothies

8

In This Chapter

- Nutritional powerhouse smoothies
- Comforting choices for balancing pH
- Sweet and fruity treats
- Versatile smoothies for alkaline meals and snacks

Smoothies are perfect foods on the pH balance diet. They pack a ton of nutrition in a quick and easy-to-drink package. Plus, they're close enough to ice cream or milkshakes, you can almost convince yourself you're indulging in these sweet treats—but without the guilt!

Filled with astonishing nutrition and near-endless possibilities for alkalizing ingredients, smoothies offer versatile choices for nourishing breakfasts, quick and convenient lunches, and anytime snacks.

Sunrise Smoothie

This smoothie is all tart and creamy nectarine-flavored goodness in a glass—yum!

Yield:	Prep time:	Serving size:	
2 smoothies	5 minutes	1 smoothie	
Each serving has:			
68.6g carbohydrate	7g fat	6.2g fiber	17.7g protein

2 medium nectarines, halved and pitted

1 cup green grapes, rinsed and stems removed

1 (8-oz.) pkg. plain yogurt

1 tsp. honey

1 TB. sunflower seeds

1. Cut nectarines into chunks that will fit into your juicer's feed tube.

2. Juice nectarines and green grapes together.

3. In a blender, process juice, yogurt, honey, and sunflower seeds until smooth and creamy.

4. Pour into glasses, and serve immediately.

BALANCE BONUS

If you like your smoothies extra cold and frosty, toss in a handful of frozen fruit chunks or several ice cubes before you blend.

Basic Strawberry Banana Smoothie

Bursting with irresistibly zingy strawberry flavor, this is one of the easiest and yummiest smoothies you can make.

Yield:	Prep time:	Serving size:	
2 smoothies	5 minutes	1 smoothie	
Each serving has:			
30g carbohydrate	3g fat	3.5g fiber	5g protein

1 cup unsweetened almond, coconut, or soy milk

1½ cups frozen strawberries

1 frozen banana, peeled and cut into 1-in. chunks

1. In a blender, process almond milk, strawberries, and banana until smooth and creamy.

2. Pour into glasses, and serve immediately.

BALANCE BONUS

Stocking up on bananas when they go on sale because they're starting to get spotty is a smart idea if you like smoothies. When you get the bananas home, peel them, cut each one into four chunks, pop them in a zipper-lock plastic bag, and freeze them. Then you'll always have some frozen bananas ready for a spur-of-the-moment smoothie break.

Velvety Banana Smoothie

Apples and yogurt brighten the richness of the banana-flavored base of this yummy drink.

Yield:	Prep time:	Serving size:	
2 smoothies	5 minutes	1 smoothie	
Each serving has:			
41.5g carbohydrate	5.1g fat	6.7g fiber	3.4g protein

2 medium apples	2 TB. plain yogurt
1 medium banana, peeled and cut into 1-in. chunks	1 TB. *tahini*
	½ tsp. sesame seeds

1. Cut apples into chunks that will fit into your juicer's feed tube, and juice apples.

2. In a blender, process apple juice, banana, yogurt, and tahini until completely smooth and frothy.

3. Pour into glasses, garnish with sesame seeds, and serve immediately.

DEFINITION

Tahini is a paste made from sesame seeds. It's used to flavor many Middle Eastern recipes.

Super Green Smoothie

This delicious smoothie relies on sweet pear juice and creamy avocado to work its alkalizing mineral magic.

Yield:	Prep time:	Serving size:	
2 smoothies	5 minutes	1 smoothie	
Each serving has:			
14.2g carbohydrate	2.5g fat	3g fiber	2.9g protein

1 medium fresh pear	½ ripe Hass avocado, peeled and seeded
¼ medium cucumber	
1 handful baby spinach leaves	½ tsp. green vegetable powder supplement (such as Kyo-Green)
4 sprigs fresh parsley	
	1 Brazil nut, grated

1. Cut pear and cucumber into chunks that will fit into your juicer's feed tube.

2. Ball up baby spinach leaves and parsley, and push them through your juicer's feed tube using pear and cucumber pieces.

3. In a blender, process juice, Hass avocado, and green vegetable powder supplement until completely smooth.

4. Pour into glasses, garnish with grated Brazil nut, and serve immediately.

BALANCE BONUS

This recipe makes a wonderfully refreshing raw chilled soup. To give it a little more pizzazz, blend in 1 or 2 teaspoons lemon juice along with the avocado.

Papaya Coconut Dream Smoothie

In this smoothie, papaya and coconut milk and oil combine to create a low-acid treat with exotic, tropical notes.

Yield:	Prep time:	Serving size:	
2 smoothies	5 minutes	1 smoothie	
Each serving has:			
18.5g carbohydrate	11.5g fat	2.7g fiber	6.3g protein

¾ cup coconut milk

1 small papaya, peeled, seeded, and cut into chunks

1 TB. virgin coconut oil

1 TB. freshly ground flaxseeds

1 tsp. vanilla extract (optional)

6 ice cubes

1. In a blender, process coconut milk, papaya, virgin coconut oil, flaxseeds, and vanilla extract (if using) until smooth and creamy.

2. Add ice cubes, and process again until smooth.

3. Pour into glasses, and serve immediately.

PHABULOUS PHACT

Papaya is a low-acid fruit that's also low on the glycemic scale, which makes it an excellent fruit for those trying to maintain a balanced pH.

Coconut Caribbean Cream Smoothie

Let the coconut and dates in this creamy smoothie transport you to your own private island oasis.

Yield:	Prep time:	Serving size:	
2 smoothies	5 minutes	1 smoothie	
Each serving has:			
15.7g carbohydrate	10.4g fat	3.8g fiber	6.1g protein

½ cup almond, coconut, or soy milk

6 oz. (about ½ block) soft tofu

⅓ cup grated coconut

3 medium dates, pitted and chopped

1 tsp. vanilla extract (optional)

6 ice cubes

1. In a blender, process almond milk, tofu, coconut, dates, vanilla extract (if using), and ice cubes on high speed until smooth.

2. Pour into glasses, and serve immediately.

PHABULOUS PHACT

Recent studies conducted at the Rambam Hospital and Technion–Israel Institute of Technology in Haifa, Israel, show that, even as sweet as they are, dates don't raise blood sugar levels appreciably. What's more, they might even aid in the prevention of atherosclerosis (hardening of the arteries).

Piña Colada Smoothie

This delicious smoothie captures all the flavors of Puerto Rico—minus the rum—in a single glass.

Yield:	Prep time:	Serving size:	
2 smoothies	5 minutes	1 smoothie	
Each serving has:			
15.8g carbohydrate	0g fat	4.5g fiber	26.2g protein

½ cup pineapple tidbits (fresh or canned in unsweetened juice)

½ cup water

1 cup coconut milk

1 cup unsweetened almond milk

2 scoops vanilla whey protein powder (or the equivalent of about 50g protein)

1 TB. freshly ground flaxseeds

6 ice cubes

1. In a blender, process pineapple tidbits and water until smooth.

2. Add coconut milk, almond milk, vanilla whey protein powder, and flaxseeds, and blend for a few more seconds or until thoroughly combined.

3. Add ice cubes, and process until ice is well incorporated and no large chunks remain.

4. Pour into glasses, and serve immediately.

BALANCE BONUS

If you really miss the flavor and fragrance of rum in your piña colada, you can add ¼ or ½ teaspoon rum-flavored extract to your smoothie without altering its pH significantly. You can find rum-flavored extract near the baking goods in most supermarkets.

Very Berry Smoothie

The alkalizing green vegetable powder supplement gives this smoothie an unusual green color, but its brisk berry flavor still comes bursting through.

Yield:	Prep time:	Serving size:	
2 smoothies	5 minutes	1 smoothie	
Each serving has:			
11.5g carbohydrate	5.1g fat	4.9g fiber	24g protein

1 cup frozen mixed berries

½ cup water

1 cup plain almond milk

2 scoops vanilla whey protein powder (or the equivalent of about 50g protein)

1 TB. green vegetable powder supplement

1 TB. freshly ground flaxseeds

3 ice cubes

1. In a blender, process mixed berries and water until smooth.

2. Add almond milk, vanilla whey protein powder, green vegetable powder supplement, and flaxseeds, and blend until thoroughly combined.

3. Add ice cubes, and process until smooth and frosty.

4. Pour into glasses, and serve immediately.

PHABULOUS PHACT

You don't really need recipes for juices or smoothies. Let your taste buds be your guide. If certain vegetables taste good together in a salad, they'll make a great juice or smoothie combo. The same thing goes for fruit. And of course, there's nothing wrong with keeping things simple by using a single fruit or vegetable on its own.

Good-Morning Grapefruit Smoothie

The vanilla whey protein powder in this recipe makes a smoothie that's reminiscent of the famous Orange Julius, but with the extra zing of grapefruit!

Yield:	Prep time:	Serving size:	
2 smoothies	5 minutes	1 smoothie	
Each serving has:			
15.8g carbohydrate	6.4g fat	4.2g fiber	24.7g protein

1 cup freshly squeezed grapefruit juice

1 cup plain almond milk

2 scoops vanilla whey protein powder (or the equivalent of about 50g protein)

1 TB. green vegetable powder supplement

1 TB. freshly ground flaxseeds

6 ice cubes

1. In a blender, process grapefruit juice, almond milk, vanilla whey protein powder, green vegetable powder supplement, and flaxseeds until smooth.

2. Add ice cubes, and blend until smooth and frosty.

3. Pour into glasses, and serve immediately.

ACID ALERT!

Be sure to check with your pharmacist before consuming grapefruit if you're taking any prescription medication. Grapefruit and grapefruit juice contain natural substances that can cause some medications to become toxic (far more powerful than they should be) or block a medicine's actions, rendering it completely ineffective.

Chocolaty Almond Butter Smoothie

There's no need to miss your favorite chocolate-almond candy bar when you can have this smoothie instead.

Yield:	Prep time:	Serving size:	
2 smoothies	5 minutes	1 smoothie	
Each serving has:			
17.1g carbohydrate	16.6g fat	4.9g fiber	26.7g protein

2½ cups plain almond milk

2 scoops vanilla whey protein powder (or the equivalent of about 50g protein)

2 TB. almond butter

2 TB. unsweetened cocoa powder

1 TB. raw cane sugar (evaporated cane juice)

3 ice cubes

1. In a blender, process almond milk, vanilla whey protein powder, almond butter, and cocoa powder until smooth.

2. Add ice cubes, and blend until smooth.

3. Pour into glasses, and serve immediately.

PHABULOUS PHACT

Scientific studies have shown that cocoa flavanols help support healthy blood circulation, as well as maintain your arteries' flexibility.

Very Veggie Smoothie

This refreshing smoothie makes a quick but flavorful pick-me-up—and also doubles as a light meal.

Yield:	Prep time:	Serving size:	
2 smoothies	5 minutes	1 smoothie	
Each serving has:			
37.4g carbohydrate	15.2g fat	14.1g fiber	3.9g protein

1 medium apple

6 medium carrots

¼ medium fresh lemon (leave peel on if organic)

8 to 10 fresh basil leaves

1 medium very ripe Hass avocado, peeled and seeded

1. Cut apple into pieces that will fit into your juicer's feed tube.

2. Ball up basil, and push it through your juicer's feed tube using carrots, apple, and lemon pieces.

3. Pour juice into a blender, add Hass avocado, and blend until smooth and creamy.

4. Pour into glasses, and serve immediately.

BALANCE BONUS

If this smoothie is too thick for you, add a little water while blending. To make it frosty, blend in a few ice cubes.

Good-Start Breakfasts

In This Chapter

- The smart way to break your fast
- Quick-fix portable breakfasts
- Unique twists on the morning meal

You've probably heard that breakfast is the most important meal of the day. After all, that first meal of the day breaks the fast your body has been in since your dinner the night before and gets your body fueled and ready for the day.

During the night, your body assimilated the nutrients you consumed during the day and rebuilt and repaired tissues. Then sometime before you woke up, it began the process of elimination, ridding the body of toxins and other bits and pieces it couldn't use. When you wake up, it's time to take in new nutrients again. You must replace the water, vitamins, and minerals your body used overnight so the cycle can continue. Yet so many people skip breakfast. And many of those who don't make poor breakfast choices.

Start every day with an alkalizing glass of warm water and a squeeze of lemon. Then try a fruit smoothie, or treat yourself to a glass of herbal tea and a bowl of quick and nourishing miso soup. A fresh bowl of berries or half a melon requires almost no prep time, and it's a sweet and refreshing way to start your day.

And don't forget about last night's leftovers. There's nothing wrong with eating grilled salmon or poached chicken in the morning. Give yourself permission to think outside the breakfast box, starting with the recipes in this chapter.

Delicious Breakfast Ideas

Breakfast can be quick and easy if you shop regularly—say, once a week—and keep fresh fruits and vegetables on hand. You can eat fresh fruits as they are, quickly juiced, or incorporated into any number of smoothies, teas, or tisanes.

Here are some good fruits to keep on hand for breakfasts and snacking:

Apples	Kiwi	Plums
Apricots	Lemons	Pomegranate
Blueberries	Mango	Raspberries
Cantaloupe	Oranges	Strawberries
Cherries	Papaya	Tangerines
Cranberries	Peaches	Watermelon
Grapefruit	Pears	
Grapes	Pineapple	

Here are some other quick and easy breakfast ideas:

- An entire tub of berries
- A bowl of mixed fruit salad topped with a dollop of plain yogurt and a sprinkle of sunflower seeds
- A large glass of your favorite fresh vegetables juiced—perfect to prepare and sip on your way to work!
- A quick smoothie (recipes in Chapter 8)
- A cup of hot water with instant miso soup stirred in

If you have more time on your hands, whip up some of the following recipes for a fantastic way to start your day.

Quick Oats

This hearty, stick-to-your-ribs oatmeal features dried fruit, fragrantly flavorful cinnamon, and coconut oil.

Yield:	Prep time:	Cook time:	Serving size:
1 cup	1 minute	2 minutes	1 cup
Each serving has:			
21.3g carbohydrate	2.3g fat	1.5g fiber	4.7g protein

⅓ cup old-fashioned rolled oats	1 tsp. virgin coconut oil
1 small handful dried apricots (diced), raisins, or cranberries	⅔ cup water
	1 sprinkle cinnamon (optional)

1. Place old-fashioned rolled oats, dried apricots, virgin coconut oil, and water in a microwave-safe bowl.

2. Cook on high for 1 or 2 minutes, watching carefully to prevent oats from boiling over.

3. Sprinkle with cinnamon (if using), stir, and serve immediately.

BALANCE BONUS

To keep your morning porridge interesting, vary your add-ins. Cacao nibs, chopped nuts, and seasonal fresh fruit are a few good choices to consider.

Savory Quinoa Breakfast Bowl

Customize this fragrant and nutty breakfast bowl with your favorite herbs.

Yield:	Prep time:	Cook time:	Serving size:
2 cups	1 minute	15 minutes	1 cup

Each serving has:			
130.6g carbohydrate	1.4g fat	29.2g fiber	31g protein

2 cups water

1 cup quinoa, rinsed and drained

Pinch sea salt

¼ tsp. parsley, chives, garlic chives, or your choice of dried herbs

Almond milk (optional)

1. In a small saucepan over medium-high heat, bring water to a boil. Stir in quinoa, sea salt, and dried herbs, and return to a boil.

2. Reduce heat to low, cover, and simmer for about 15 minutes or until ¾ of water has absorbed.

3. Serve hot, topped with a little almond milk (if using).

PHABULOUS PHACT

Ordinary culinary herbs offer many health benefits. Chief among many herbs' benefits are their ability to aid proper digestion and their high nutritional value. Experiment and use them generously in all your food preparations.

Easy Leftover Brown Rice Pudding

Turn leftover brown rice into a breakfast treat flavored with almonds and soft, warm raisins.

Yield:	Prep time:	Cook time:	Serving size:
3 cups	5 minutes	15 minutes	1 cup

Each serving has:			
120.7g carbohydrate	24.5g fat	7.2g fiber	12.6g protein

2 cups cooked brown rice	½ tsp. ground cinnamon
1 cup almond milk	½ tsp. pure organic vanilla extract
¼ cup raisins	
2 TB. sliced almonds	2 TB. pure maple syrup

1. In a medium saucepan over medium-high heat, combine brown rice, almond milk, raisins, almonds, cinnamon, vanilla extract, and maple syrup. Bring to a boil.

2. Reduce heat to medium, and cook, stirring frequently, for about 15 minutes or until rice is thick and creamy.

3. Serve immediately.

BALANCE BONUS

Freeze or refrigerate leftover grains and even beans in zipper-lock plastic bags, and use them for quick and easy additions to soups, casseroles, and other dishes.

Spelt Berry Porridge

Spelt berries are wonderfully chewy and nutty, and in this recipe, they're complemented by the comforting combination of apples, vanilla, and cinnamon.

Yield:	Prep time:	Cook time:	Serving size:
8 cups	5 minutes	45 minutes	1 cup

Each serving has:			
81.5g carbohydrate	2g fat	14.5g fiber	10g protein

2 cups *spelt* berries	2 apples, cored and roughly chopped
6 cups water	
2 tsp. pure organic vanilla extract	½ cup walnuts, chopped
½ tsp. ground cinnamon	Kefir or plain yogurt (optional)

1. Rinse spelt berries several times, drain, and set aside.

2. In a medium saucepan over medium-high heat, bring water to a boil. Add spelt berries, reduce heat to medium-low, cover, and cook for about 45 minutes or until spelt berries are tender.

3. Stir in vanilla extract, cinnamon, and apples.

4. Top each serving with 1 tablespoon walnuts and 1 tablespoon kefir (if using), and serve hot.

DEFINITION

Spelt berries are an ancient type of wheat originally grown around 5000 to 6000 B.C.E. in what's now Iran. They're valued for their nutty flavor and high protein and nutrition content. Note that spelt does contain gluten.

Breakfast Biscuits with Smoked Salmon

The salmon contributes its smoky flavor to these biscuits, making them reminiscent of the classic combo lox and bagels.

Yield:	Prep time:	Cook time:	Serving size:
8 biscuits	10 minutes	12 minutes	2 biscuits

Each serving has:			
46.9g carbohydrate	11g fat	7.7g fiber	9.8g protein

2 green onions, white and green parts, finely chopped	2 cups spelt flour
2 TB. smoked salmon, finely diced	1½ TB. baking powder
1 tsp. fresh dill weed, chopped	¼ tsp. sea salt
	3 TB. ghee or butter
	1 cup water

1. Preheat the oven to 425°F. Lightly coat a baking sheet with cooking spray, and set aside.

2. In a small bowl, toss together green onions, smoked salmon, dill weed, and 1 tablespoon spelt flour.

3. In a large bowl, stir together remaining spelt flour, baking powder, and sea salt.

4. Add salmon mixture to the large bowl, and stir until well incorporated.

5. Using a fork or a pastry cutter, cut ghee and water into flour mixture, and stir to create a thick batter.

6. Spoon 8 equal-size mounds of batter onto the prepared baking sheet, leaving plenty of room for biscuits to expand, and bake for 12 minutes.

7. Serve warm as is, or split and spread with a little light cream cheese.

DEFINITION

Ghee is a clarified butter used extensively in Indian cuisine. After the milk solids and water are removed, only pure butterfat remains. In fact, the word *ghee* is the Hindi word for "fat."

Perky Pumpkin Pancakes

The harvest-time flavor and aroma of these pumpkin pancakes add a warm sweetness to your morning meal.

Yield:	Prep time:	Cook time:	Serving size:
8 pancakes	10 minutes	20 minutes	2 pancakes

Each serving has:			
41.6g carbohydrate	11.6g fat	5.9g fiber	6g protein

½ cup canned organic pumpkin purée

¾ cup almond milk

¼ cup water

¼ cup organic unrefined cane sugar (sucanat or evaporated cane juice)

1 TB. ghee

½ tsp. pumpkin pie spices (ginger, cinnamon, cloves)

1 TB. orange zest

2 tsp. grated ginger

¼ tsp. sea salt

½ cup kamut flour

½ cup spelt flour

1 TB. baking powder

1. In a large bowl, stir together pumpkin purée, almond milk, water, unrefined cane sugar, ghee, pumpkin pie spices, orange zest, ginger, and sea salt. Set aside.

2. In a medium bowl, stir together kamut flour, spelt flour, and baking powder.

3. Beat flour mixture into liquid mixture a little at a time until just combined.

4. Spray a medium skillet or a griddle with cooking spray, and heat to medium-high.

5. Using a ¼-cup measure, scoop batter onto the hot skillet, and cook for about 2 minutes or until edges are dry and center is bubbly.

6. Using a spatula, turn over pancakes and cook for about 1 more minute or until cooked through and nicely browned on both sides. Repeat with remaining batter, and serve warm.

South-of-the-Border Breakfast Burritos

Brimming with the mouthwatering Mexican flavors of sweet red and green peppers, fresh cilantro, queso fresco, and tomato salsa, these burritos are perfect for a leisurely Sunday brunch.

Yield:	Prep time:	Cook time:	Serving size:
4 burritos	15 minutes	15 minutes	1 burrito
Each serving has:			
33.7g carbohydrate	13.5g fat	7.8g fiber	16.3g protein

1 TB. olive oil	¼ cup fresh cilantro, minced
1 medium yellow onion, finely chopped	½ tsp. sea salt
1 medium green bell pepper, ribs and seeds removed, and chopped	4 large organic free-range eggs, beaten
	4 large sprouted whole-grain tortillas
1 medium red bell pepper, ribs and seeds removed, and chopped	¼ cup shredded *queso fresco*
	4 TB. prepared organic tomato salsa
1 small zucchini, diced	

1. In a large, heavy skillet over medium heat, heat olive oil. Add onion, green bell pepper, red bell pepper, and zucchini, and sauté for about 5 minutes or until tender-crisp.

2. Sprinkle with cilantro and sea salt, and sauté for 1 more minute.

3. Pour beaten eggs over vegetables, and when bottom and edges of eggs begin to set, use a spatula to gently pull egg mixture back and forth across the skillet until all eggs are set.

4. Divide egg mixture into equal portions and spoon in a line down center of each whole-grain tortilla. Top with equal portions of queso fresco and tomato salsa, roll tortilla into a log, and serve warm.

PHABULOUS PHACT

Eggs are not an alkalizing food, but they are an important source of many nutrients and shouldn't be excluded from a healthy diet. On days when you eat eggs, balance your diet with an abundance of vegetables and fresh leafy greens.

Lunch Box Best Bets

In This Chapter

- Planning for lunchtime success
- New recipes to keep lunch interesting
- Making meal prep easier

It's easy to allow lunchtime to turn into I'm-in-a-hurry-so-I'll-grab-whatever's-convenient-whether-it's-necessarily-healthy-or-not-time, which can quickly derail your best dietary plans. But with only a little advance planning, you can whip up delicious pH balance diet–friendly lunches that will keep you on track and in balance.

This chapter offers several tasty lunch ideas. All are easy to create and can be prepared ahead of time if mornings don't hold a lot of extra time for you. Keeping a few standard ingredients such as precooked beans or grains and prepped fruits and vegetables ready in your refrigerator or freezer helps make meal preparations even easier.

Veggie Burgers

These vegetarian burgers are bean based and flavored with fresh herbs and savory *miso broth*.

Yield:	Prep time:	Cook time:	Serving size:
4 burgers	6 minutes	30 minutes	1 burger

Each serving has:			
28.2g carbohydrate	0.9g fat	3.8g fiber	3.5g protein

2 cups your choice cooked dried beans

1 cup steamed winter squash

1 medium carrot, grated

1 small shallot, minced

½ cup cooked brown rice

1 TB. your choice fresh herbs, finely chopped, or 1 tsp. dried

½ cup miso broth

Avocado Cream Sauce (recipe in Chapter 12)

2 TB. sesame, hemp, or sunflower seeds

1. Preheat the oven to 350°F.

2. Place beans in a large bowl and, using a fork, mash well.

3. Add winter squash, carrot, shallot, brown rice, and herbs, and mix well. Add miso broth a little at a time, and mix well.

4. Form into 4 patties, place on a nonstick baking sheet, and bake for 30 minutes.

5. Serve warm or at room temperature topped with Avocado Cream Sauce and garnished with sesame, hemp, or sunflower seeds.

Variation: Many other herbs or spices work nicely in these burgers. Try basil, cumin, dill, garlic, ginger, fennel, mint, parsley, sage, or thyme.

DEFINITION

Miso broth is made from miso paste, a thick, salty, tangy base composed of fermented soybeans, barley, rice, or other grains commonly used in Japanese-style soups. It also adds a unique flavor to salad dressings, sauces and marinades, baked tofu, or vegetable dishes.

Tabbouleh Wraps

You'll fall in love with the bright mint, fresh parsley, and cucumber flavors of this easy Middle Eastern–style meal.

Yield:	Prep time:	Serving size:
4 wraps	25 minutes	1 wrap

Each serving has:			
26.4g carbohydrate	5.6g fat	5.1g fiber	6.1g protein

²⁄₃ cup cooked quinoa

½ cup fresh mint, chopped

1½ cups fresh parsley, chopped

1 large ripe tomato, diced

1 medium cucumber, diced (peeled, if not organic)

⅓ cup green onion, white and green parts, sliced

1 TB. extra-virgin olive oil

Juice of 1 lemon

Pinch sea salt

4 large leaves romaine lettuce

1 medium lemon, quartered into wedges

1. In a large bowl, combine quinoa, mint, parsley, tomato, cucumber, green onion, extra-virgin olive oil, lemon juice, and sea salt. Cover and refrigerate for 20 minutes to let flavors meld.

2. Evenly divide tabbouleh among romaine lettuce leaves, and mound along central stem. Roll leaf into a log, and secure with a toothpick.

3. Serve wraps cold or at room temperature with a wedge of lemon.

DEFINITION

Tabbouleh is a traditional Arabian salad made of bulgur wheat, chopped tomatoes, parsley, mint, onion, and garlic, and marinated in a dressing of olive oil, lemon juice, and salt. Western variations include tabbouleh dishes made with couscous or quinoa instead of cracked wheat. This version uses quinoa instead of bulgur wheat to make it a little more pH friendly.

White Bean Salad

Hearty navy beans are the basis of this veggie-rich salad that features the zing of healthful, naturally made pickles and sauerkraut.

Yield:	Prep time:	Serving size:	
4 main-dish salads	5 minutes	1 salad	
Each serving has:			
40.7g carbohydrate	1.1g fat	14.6g fiber	14.1g protein

1 (15-oz.) can organic, no-salt-added navy beans, rinsed and drained

1 medium celery rib, finely chopped

3 medium naturally fermented dill gherkins, finely chopped

1 medium red bell pepper, ribs and seeds removed, and sliced

1 medium yellow bell pepper, ribs and seeds removed, and sliced

4 cups mixed salad greens

$\frac{1}{2}$ cup naturally fermented sauerkraut, rinsed and drained

2 TB. sunflower seeds

Lively Lime Vinaigrette (recipe in Chapter 11)

1. In a large bowl, toss navy beans, celery, dill gherkins, red bell pepper, yellow bell pepper, mixed salad greens, and sauerkraut.

2. Divide among 4 large individual salad plates, garnish with sunflower seeds, and drizzle on some Lively Lime Vinaigrette (recipe in Chapter 11) or another light vinaigrette dressing.

PHABULOUS PHACT

If you don't make your own lacto-fermented pickles and sauerkraut, you can often find them in the refrigerator section of your supermarket. Lacto-fermented vegetables are far superior to other pickles that have been processed in vinegar and pasteurized. Like yogurt, lacto-fermented vegetables contain live probiotic cultures and active enzymes, and they retain a high level of vitamin and mineral content.

Leafy Tuna Lunch

Mixed baby greens provide a nice balance of sweet, earthy, and bitter flavors as a backdrop to the fish and fresh garden veggies in this lunch salad.

Yield:	Prep time:	Serving size:	
1 main-dish salad	5 minutes	1 salad	
Each serving has:			
33.6g carbohydrate	4.6g fat	9.1g fiber	47.3g protein

1 (5- or 6-oz.) bag organic mixed baby salad greens

1 (6-oz.) can tuna steak in spring water, drained

6 grape tomatoes, cut in half

$\frac{1}{2}$ medium cucumber, sliced (peeled if not organic)

1 TB. fresh dill weed, chopped

1 wedge lemon

1. Place baby salad greens on a large salad plate.

2. Flake tuna steak using a fork, and arrange on top of salad greens. Top with grape tomatoes, cucumber slices, and dill weed.

3. Squeeze lemon wedge over salad, and enjoy.

PHABULOUS PHACT

Dill weed is an excellent source of vitamin C and pro-vitamin A, as well as minerals like potassium, calcium, manganese, and magnesium. Potassium is an important component of cell and body fluids that helps control heart rate and blood pressure. Your body uses manganese as a co-factor (a type of molecule that helps enzymes carry out chemical reactions) for the antioxidant enzyme superoxide dismutase.

Beet Salad with Sweet Potato

This lunch salad is a perfect balance of naturally sweet roasted sweet potatoes served alongside a zingy marinated beet salad. It's best prepared the night before.

Yield:	Prep time:	Cook time:	Serving size:
1 sweet potato and side salad	10 minutes, plus overnight	55 to 70 minutes	1 sweet potato and salad

Each serving has:			
89.4g carbohydrate	5.7g fat	21.1g fiber	14.9g protein

1 large sweet potato, scrubbed

1 lb. baby beets, scrubbed and trimmed

½ medium cucumber, sliced

1 medium green onion, white and green parts, sliced

1 TB. sesame seeds

Handful alfalfa sprouts

1 TB. apple cider vinegar

1. Preheat the oven to 450°F. Line a baking sheet with aluminum foil.

2. Place sweet potato on the prepared baking sheet, and bake for 45 minutes to 1 hour or until potato's skin is loose and some syrup has oozed out and charred on the foil. Reserve potato at room temperature in the oven, or in the refrigerator, overnight.

3. Meanwhile, place beets in a steamer, and steam for 7 to 10 minutes or until tender-crisp.

4. When beets have cooled enough to be handled, slice and place in a nonmetallic bowl.

5. Add cucumber, green onion, sesame seeds, and alfalfa sprouts. Top with apple cider vinegar, and stir to coat. Cover salad, and refrigerate overnight.

6. In the morning, pack your prepared salad and potato, and go!

Tuna Steak with Kale and Caper Dressing

Meaty tuna steak and super-alkalizing kale make a hearty lunch. Salty capers and tangy rice wine vinegar balance the earthy flavors of the greens and chickpeas.

Yield:	Prep time:	Cook time:	Serving size:
1 tuna steak with greens	10 minutes	10 minutes	1 tuna steak with greens

Each serving has:			
123.3g carbohydrate	27.7g fat	36g fiber	90.4g protein

1 (6-oz.) fresh tuna steak	3 TB. fresh parsley, chopped
2 TB. water	Juice of 1 medium lemon
Large handful fresh kale (about $\frac{1}{3}$ lb.), stems removed and roughly chopped	1 tsp. extra-virgin olive oil
	3 TB. hot water
	1 cup cooked chickpeas
3 TB. capers	1 TB. rice wine vinegar

1. In a hot skillet over high heat, cook tuna steak for about 2 or 3 minutes per side or until desired doneness. Remove tuna steak, and set aside.

2. Add water and kale to the skillet, and sauté kale for about 2 minutes or until wilted but still bright green. Remove from heat.

3. In a glass jar with a lid, add capers, parsley, lemon juice, extra-virgin olive oil, and hot water. Screw on the lid and shake vigorously for a few seconds to combine. Set aside.

4. In a blender, process chickpeas and rice wine vinegar until smooth.

5. Spoon blended chickpeas in an even layer on a plate. Top with tuna steak, and arrange kale on the side. Pour half of caper dressing over all, and serve warm or at room temperature.

Variation: If chickpeas aren't your favorite, replace them with $\frac{1}{2}$ ripe Hass avocado, sliced, and a squeeze of lemon juice.

Quick Quinoa Bowl

Nutty quinoa packs a high-fiber protein punch that will keep your hunger in check until late in the day. Green beans, cucumber, sweet bell peppers, and cherry tomatoes define the garden-fresh flavors of this dish.

Yield:	Prep time:	Cook time:	Serving size:
4 grain and veggie bowls	10 minutes	20 minutes	1 bowl

Each serving has:			
32.4g carbohydrate	9.1g fat	6.1g fiber	6.8g protein

½ cup uncooked quinoa	6 cherry tomatoes, halved
1 cup fresh or frozen green beans, cut into 1-in. pieces	2 TB. olive oil
½ medium cucumber, thinly sliced (peeled if not organic)	2 TB. freshly squeezed lemon juice
½ medium yellow bell pepper, ribs and seeds removed, and thinly sliced	1 clove garlic, crushed and minced
	2 TB. fresh parsley, minced

1. In a medium saucepan over medium-high heat, prepare quinoa according to package instructions. Drain quinoa in a colander under cool running water, and gently press quinoa against the colander to remove excess moisture. Place quinoa in a large bowl, and set aside.

2. In a small pan over medium-high heat, cook green beans in boiling water for about 5 minutes or until tender-crisp. Drain beans in the colander and cool quickly under cool running water.

3. Add green beans, cucumber, yellow bell pepper, cherry tomatoes, olive oil, lemon juice, garlic, and parsley to the bowl with quinoa, and stir well.

4. Allow mixture to sit, covered, for 15 minutes or more before serving.

Cashew Tofu Toss for Two

Salty tamari, nutty cashews, and stir-fried garden vegetables come together to create this pH-balancing, easy-to-pack Asian-inspired lunch.

Yield:	Prep time:	Cook time:	Serving size:
2 salads	10 minutes	5 minutes	1 salad
Each serving has:			
18.2g carbohydrate	13.6g fat	5.5g fiber	7.4g protein

1 TB. olive oil

1 medium red bell pepper, ribs and seeds removed, and cut into 1-in. squares

1 cup snow peas, trimmed and cut into thirds

1 heart romaine lettuce

1 tsp. wheat-free tamari sauce

4 oz. (about ⅓ carton) firm tofu, cut into ½-in. cubes

2 medium green onions, white and green parts, sliced

¼ cup plain cashews, roughly chopped

Additional olive oil and tamari

1. In a wok or a large skillet over medium heat, heat olive oil. Add red bell pepper, and stir-fry for 2 or 3 minutes or until tender-crisp.

2. Add snow peas, and cook for 30 more seconds.

3. Separate romaine lettuce leaves, tear into bite-size pieces, and divide evenly between 2 large salad plates. Arrange tofu cubes on lettuce, garnish with green onions and cashews, drizzle with additional tamari and olive oil to taste, and serve.

BALANCE BONUS

This recipe is just as tasty with lemony chicken breast or whitefish in place of the tofu.

Nummy Nutty Pâté

Brazil nuts and cashews create a richly satisfying protein-rich pâté, perfect alongside a variety of fresh vegetables.

Yield:	Prep time:	Serving size:	
1 cup	5 minutes	1/2 cup	
Each serving has:			
19.5g carbohydrate	62g fat	4.1g fiber	15.7g protein

½ cup raw Brazil nuts, roughly chopped

½ cup raw cashews, roughly chopped

2 tsp. extra-virgin olive oil

1 clove garlic, crushed and minced

1 TB. freshly squeezed lemon juice

½ cup chopped fresh parsley

¼ cup cold water

1. In a food processor fitted with a chopping blade or in a blender, process Brazil nuts, cashews, extra-virgin olive oil, garlic, lemon juice, parsley, and cold water until almost completely smooth. Some chunks and bits of nuts will remain.

2. Serve with a variety of fresh vegetables such as carrot sticks, broccoli and cauliflower florets, celery sticks, and bell pepper strips.

3. Refrigerate leftover pâté in an airtight container for up to 2 days.

PHABULOUS PHACT

Fresh lemon juice is highly alkalizing. Add it to plain water or teas, and use it to brighten the flavor of seafood, pork, chicken, and vegetables while decreasing the acidity of your meals at the same time.

Herb-Roasted Cod and Veggies

Oregano, rosemary, and basil shine in this easy veggie-and-seafood lunch with an Italian flair.

Yield:	Prep time:	Cook time:	Serving size:
2 cod fillets and veggies	10 minutes	40 minutes	1 cod fillet and veggies

Each serving has:			
12g carbohydrate	16.1g fat	4g fiber	41.1g protein

2 (4- to 6-oz.) cod fillets

1 tsp. Italian seasoning

2 medium ripe tomatoes, sliced

2 medium zucchini, cut into $\frac{1}{2}$-in. chunks

1 medium red bell pepper, ribs and seeds removed, and cut into 1-in. squares

1 medium yellow bell pepper, ribs and seeds removed, and cut into 1-inch squares

4 shallots, peeled and halved or quartered vertically

2 TB. olive oil

1. Preheat the oven to 350°F.

2. Place each cod fillet on one side of a sheet of parchment paper or aluminum foil large enough to enclose fish like an envelope.

3. Sprinkle $\frac{1}{2}$ teaspoon Italian seasoning over cod, top fillets with several tomato slices, and sprinkle remaining $\frac{1}{2}$ teaspoon Italian seasoning over tomatoes.

4. Bring free edge of the parchment paper up and over the cod so the upper and lower edges meet. Beginning on one open corner, firmly crease and fold the paper all the way around the three open edges until cod is completely encased.

5. Place zucchini, red bell pepper, yellow bell pepper, and shallots on a large baking sheet. Drizzle with olive oil, and toss lightly to coat.

6. Place cod packets next to vegetables on the baking sheet, and bake for 15 minutes.

7. Remove cod packets from the baking sheet, set aside, and keep warm. Return vegetables to the oven and cook for 20 more minutes or until just tender and lightly browned.

8. Place 1 cod packet on each of 2 plates. Slit open the parchment paper and serve fish accompanied by half the roasted vegetables.

BALANCE BONUS

Balancing your diet's pH doesn't mean eating everything raw or even only plant-based food. It only means choosing more vegetables than fruit and going light on meats. Place more of your dietary emphasis on leafy green vegetables, and steer clear of sugar and processed or artificial ingredients.

Sensational Salads and Dressings

In This Chapter

- Discovering new salad ingredients
- Quick and easy salads
- Exploring pH balance salads and dressings

It shouldn't surprise you to see a salad chapter in a diet book. But rest assured, the salads in this chapter are so much more than the same old iceberg lettuce with a slice of tomato on top. As you'll see in these pages, you can create unique fruit-and-vegetable combinations, use mineral-rich sea vegetables, or even make a warm salad with grains. Because of the inherent alkalizing properties of vegetables and fruits, salads should figure prominently in your pH balance eating regimen.

To ensure you can put together a salad at a moment's notice when hunger hits, it helps to prep about 2 days' worth of simple raw salad ingredients and store them in your refrigerator. Make up a few containers of fruits and vegetables to mix in, too, such as julienned carrots, sliced cucumbers, sliced sweet peppers, and grape tomatoes. Then you can grab some salad ingredients; add some prepared fruits or vegetables; top with dressing and some nuts, seeds, or sprouts; and have a perfect salad ready to pack and go in no time!

Hiziki Salad

Hiziki (sometimes spelled *hijiki*), a Japanese sea vegetable, adds Asian flair to this alkalizing salad made with fruits like apple and cherry and ripe tomatoes and cucumber.

Yield:	Prep time:	Cook time:	Serving size:
4 side salads	10 minutes	15 minutes	1 side salad

Each serving has:			
21.4g carbohydrate	3g fat	2.8g fiber	1.6g protein

¼ cup dried hiziki	1 medium cucumber
1 cup cold water	¼ cup your choice apple, diced
1 cup water	½ cup dried cherries
4 cups baby salad greens	¼ cup sliced raw almonds
1 medium tomato, sliced	

1. In a medium bowl, soak hiziki in 1 cup cold water for 10 minutes. Drain.

2. In a small saucepan over medium heat, add soaked hiziki and 1 cup water, and bring to a simmer for 15 minutes. Drain.

3. In a large bowl, toss together baby salad greens, tomato, cucumber, apple, cherries, and hiziki.

4. Serve, topped with your favorite salad dressing and a sprinkle of sliced raw almonds.

PHABULOUS PHACT

Hiziki is one of the most highly prized Japanese sea vegetables, boasting a mild flavor and tiny, tightly wound black curls. Hiziki is washed, steamed, and dried before packaging, and it expands to about four times its dried size when soaked and cooked.

Italian-Style Three-Bean Salad

This pleasantly tangy three-bean salad packs the added nutritional punch of fresh dandelion greens and health-giving *umeboshi paste*.

Yield:	Prep time:	Cook time:	Serving size:
5 cups	10 minutes, plus 8 hours marinate time	10 minutes	$\frac{1}{2}$ cup

Each serving has:			
14g carbohydrate	1g fat	5g fiber	5g protein

1 cup cooked kidney beans, drained if canned

1 cup cooked chickpeas, drained if canned

1 cup cooked pinto beans, drained if canned

$2\frac{1}{2}$ cups water

1 cup fresh green beans, stems removed, and chopped into $\frac{1}{2}$-in. pieces

1 cup dandelion greens, washed well and coarsely chopped

1 tsp. olive oil

1 TB. umeboshi paste

$\frac{1}{4}$ cup fresh parsley, minced

$\frac{1}{4}$ cup red onion, finely chopped

2 tsp. apple cider vinegar

1. In a large, nonmetallic bowl, place kidney beans, chickpeas, and pinto beans. Set aside.

2. In a medium saucepan over medium-high heat, bring 2 cups water to a boil. Add green beans, and blanch for 3 minutes. Using a slotted spoon, remove green beans from water and place in the large bowl.

3. Add dandelion greens to boiling water in the saucepan, and blanch for 30 seconds. Drain dandelion greens and set aside.

4. In a small skillet over medium heat, heat olive oil. Add dandelion greens, and sauté for 2 minutes or until thoroughly warmed through.

5. Transfer dandelion greens to the large bowl, and toss with beans to mix. Set aside.

6. In a blender or a food processor fitted with a chopping blade, purée umeboshi paste, parsley, red onion, remaining $\frac{1}{2}$ cup water, and apple cider vinegar.

7. Pour purée over beans and dandelion greens, and stir to thoroughly combine.

8. Cover the bowl with plastic wrap, and refrigerate 8 hours or overnight.

9. Remove salad from the refrigerator, stir, and serve chilled.

DEFINITION

Umeboshi paste is a seasoning paste made of pickled Japanese ume fruit, a type of plum. The paste is salty and has a sour flavor due to its high citric acid content.

Alkalizing Apple-Cucumber Salad

This light salad, with the bright, crisp flavors of apple and cucumber, is great to eat on a hot summer day and provides balance to a heavier meal.

Yield:	Prep time:	Serving size:	
2 cups	70 minutes	1/2 cup	
Each serving has:			
9g carbohydrate	1g fat	2g fiber	1g protein

1 medium cucumber, thinly sliced

1 cup red apple, thinly sliced

2 tsp. dried wakame flakes

$1\frac{1}{2}$ TB. genmai (brown rice) miso paste

1 TB. mirin

2 tsp. brown rice vinegar

1 TB. fresh parsley, minced

$\frac{1}{2}$ cup water

2 TB. freshly squeezed orange juice

1. In a medium, nonmetallic bowl, place cucumber and red apple.

2. In a small bowl, place wakame flakes and enough cold water to cover, and soak for 10 minutes. Drain, and place wakame flakes in the medium bowl. Set aside.

3. In a blender, place genmai miso paste, mirin, brown rice vinegar, parsley, water, and orange juice, and purée until smooth and creamy.

4. Pour dressing over salad mixture, and stir to thoroughly combine.

5. Cover the bowl with plastic wrap, and place in the refrigerator to marinate for 1 hour.

6. Remove salad from the refrigerator, strain off and discard marinade, and serve chilled on individual salad plates.

DEFINITION

Mirin is a sweetish Japanese rice wine—sweeter than sake. You can find mirin in the Asian foods section of larger supermarkets, in health food stores, and online.

Greek Lentil and Fresh Dill Salad

Tangy lemon juice and fresh dill accompany crisp bits of red onion and radish in bringing this warm lentil salad to life.

Yield:	Prep time:	Cook time:	Serving size:
8 cups greens, 4 cups lentil mixture	10 minutes	15 minutes	2 cups greens, 1 cup lentil mixture

Each serving has:			
30g carbohydrate	7g fat	10g fiber	15g protein

2 TB. extra-virgin olive oil	2 TB. freshly squeezed lemon juice
3 cloves garlic, minced	$\frac{1}{8}$ tsp. freshly ground black pepper
3 medium bay leaves	
2 (15-oz.) cans Eden Organic Lentils with Onion and Bay Leaf, undrained	$\frac{1}{3}$ cup red radishes, finely sliced
	$\frac{1}{3}$ cup red onion, minced
1 cup carrots, diced	2 TB. fresh dill, minced
$\frac{1}{2}$ cup celery, finely diced	8 cups mixed baby salad greens

1. In a medium skillet over medium heat, heat extra-virgin olive oil. Add garlic, and sauté for 1 minute or until softened but not brown.

2. Add bay leaves, Eden Organic Lentils with Onion and Bay Leaf, carrots, celery, 1 tablespoon lemon juice, and black pepper, and bring to a boil.

3. Reduce heat, and simmer about 10 minutes or until vegetables are tender and about half of liquid has evaporated. Set aside and cool slightly.

4. Add red radishes, remaining 1 tablespoon lemon juice, red onion, and dill, and mix.

5. Place in a medium bowl, and toss to cool lentil mixture a bit more.

6. Evenly divide baby salad greens onto individual plates, and spoon lentil mixture over them.

7. Garnish each plate with fresh dill, and serve immediately.

BALANCE BONUS

To make this a more appealing option in warm-weather months, you can chill the Greek lentil bean mixture in the refrigerator before serving.

Jamaican Bean and Veggie Salad

The flavors and aromas of the Caribbean define this salad, composed of unusual and fresh flavor combinations like shredded coconut and dry-roasted peanuts.

Yield:	Prep time:	Serving size:	
12 cups	2 or 3 hours	2 cups	
Each serving has:			
32g carbohydrate	21g fat	10g fiber	10g protein

½ cup extra-virgin olive oil

2 cloves garlic, finely minced

1 TB. organic barley malt syrup

1 TB. organic maple syrup

1 TB. naturally fermented shoyu soy sauce

Juice of 1 lime

½ tsp. freshly ground black pepper

1 (15-oz.) can organic black-eyed peas, rinsed and drained, or 3 cups cooked dry beans

1 (15-oz.) can organic kidney beans, rinsed and drained, or 3 cups cooked dry beans

½ medium red bell pepper, ribs and seeds removed, and sliced

½ medium green bell pepper, ribs and seeds removed, and sliced

½ medium yellow bell pepper, ribs and seeds removed, and sliced

1 medium red onion, finely sliced into thin rings

2 TB. seedless raisins

2 TB. unsweetened shredded coconut

2 TB. unsalted dry-roasted peanuts (or other nuts of choice)

1. In a blender, place extra-virgin olive oil, garlic, barley malt syrup, maple syrup, shoyu soy sauce, lime juice, and black pepper, and process several seconds or until well combined. Set aside.

2. In a large bowl, combine black-eyed peas, kidney beans, red bell pepper, green bell pepper, yellow bell pepper, and red onion.

3. Add raisins, shredded coconut, and roasted peanuts, and distribute throughout.

4. Pour marinade over bean-and-vegetable mixture, and stir well. Cover, and allow to marinate for 2 or 3 hours before serving.

BALANCE BONUS

To make this salad large enough to feed a crowd, stir in organic spelt or any other whole-grain (but not wheat) pasta and serve on a generous bed of mixed spring greens.

Warm Red Lentil Salad

Fresh ginger, mint, and citrus give this warm salad a refreshingly flavorful edge.

Yield:	Prep time:	Cook time:	Serving size:
4 side or light-lunch salads	5 minutes	25 minutes	1 salad

Each serving has:			
45.8g carbohydrate	0.7g fat	26.7g fiber	17.5g protein

½ lb. split red lentils, rinsed, sorted, and dried

3 TB. onion, finely chopped

2 cloves garlic, crushed and minced

1 TB. fresh ginger, minced

1 cube vegan vegetable bouillon with sea salt and herbs (such as Rapunzel's)

1 TB. fresh mint leaves, minced (or 1 tsp. dried)

½ lb. mixed spring salad greens

8 fresh lemon or lime wedges

1. In a medium saucepan, combine split red lentils, onion, garlic, ginger, vegan vegetable bouillon cube, and mint.

3. Cover lentils with water by at least 1 inch, and bring to a boil over medium heat. Cover, and reduce heat to medium-low.

4. Allow lentils to simmer for about 25 minutes or until tender, stirring occasionally. If water level reduces by too much before lentils are tender, add more water and continue to cook a little longer.

5. Drain lentils, and serve warm on a generous bed of mixed spring salad greens with a fresh squeeze of lemon.

> **PHANTASTIC PHACT**
>
> This salad is a nutritional powerhouse—it's very low in saturated fat, cholesterol, and sodium. It's also a good source of dietary fiber, protein, vitamin C, thiamin, iron, and copper and an excellent source of vitamin A, vitamin K, folate, and manganese.

Lively Lime Vinaigrette

Freshly pressed garlic and garden herbs combine with tangy ume plum vinegar and lime in this lively salad dressing.

Yield:	Prep time:	Serving size:	
1 pint	65 minutes	1 tablespoon	
Each serving has:			
1g carbohydrate	5g fat	0g fiber	0g protein

1/3 cup extra-virgin olive oil

1/3 cup organic brown rice vinegar

1/3 cup freshly squeezed lime juice

3 TB. ume plum vinegar

2 cloves garlic, pressed

1/4 tsp. sea salt

1 TB. fresh basil, minced

1 tsp. dried basil

1 TB. fresh dill, minced

1 tsp. dried dill

3 TB. warm water

1. In a 1-quart glass jar, add extra-virgin olive oil, brown rice vinegar, lime juice, ume plum vinegar, garlic, sea salt, fresh basil, dried basil, fresh dill, dried dill, and warm water.

2. Secure the lid on the jar, and shake vigorously for 30 seconds.

3. Store covered in the refrigerator for 1 hour to chill and to allow flavors to meld.

4. Shake again before using, and serve.

BALANCE BONUS

Japanese ume products—such as ume plum vinegar, umeboshi plums, and umeboshi paste—can be found online, in most Asian food markets, and in many health-food stores.

Ginger Orange Tahini Salad Dressing

Enliven the flavors of ho-hum salad greens with bright and tangy orange juice, earthy tahini, and zippy ginger.

Yield:	Prep time:	Serving size:	
1 cup	5 minutes	2 tablespoons	
Each serving has:			
6g carbohydrate	5g fat	1g fiber	3g protein

3 TB. organic *shiro miso paste*

3 TB. organic roasted tahini

1 tsp. brown mustard

1 tsp. organic brown rice vinegar

¼ cup freshly squeezed orange juice

1 TB. fresh parsley, minced

¼ cup water

1 tsp. finely grated ginger

1. In a blender or food processor fitted with a chopping blade, process shiro miso paste, tahini, brown mustard, brown rice vinegar, orange juice, parsley, water, and ginger until smooth.

2. Serve spooned over salad greens or as a light dip for sliced vegetables.

DEFINITION

Shiro miso paste is a light yellow paste commonly known as "white miso" in the West or "summer miso" in Japan. It's less salty and undergoes a shorter fermentation period than other misos. **Tahini** is a ground sesame seed paste, similar to peanut butter, that's rich in calcium.

Garlic and Lemon Tahini Dressing

Fresh parsley brightens the earthiness of tahini as it marries perfectly with garlic and freshly squeezed lemon in this dressing.

Yield:	Prep time:	Serving size:	
⅔ cup	5 minutes	1 tablespoon	
Each serving has:			
7g carbohydrate	12g fat	2g fiber	5g protein

6 TB. organic tahini	2 TB. finely grated onion
2 TB. freshly squeezed lemon juice	½ tsp. sea salt
1 clove garlic, pressed	1 TB. fresh parsley, finely minced
	½ cup cold water

1. In a blender or food processor fitted with a chopping blade, process tahini, lemon juice, garlic, onion, sea salt, parsley, and cold water for about 30 seconds.

2. Pour into a glass canning jar with a lid, screw on the lid, and refrigerate until ready to use.

PHABULOUS PHACT

Garlic is a phenomenal superfood that may help prevent ulcers by inhibiting the growth of *Helicobacter pylori* bacteria in the stomach. Additionally, it has been shown to improve immune function and blood circulation, lower blood pressure and cholesterol, and stabilize blood sugar. Garlic's nutrients include calcium, folate, iron, magnesium, manganese, phosphorus, potassium, selenium, zinc, vitamin C, and vitamins B_1, B_2, and B_3.

Garlic Lover's Dressing

This is a dressing for true garlic lovers. If you can't get enough of the taste of garlic, you won't be able to get enough of this.

Yield:	Prep time:	Serving size:	
¼ cup	8 to 10 minutes	2 tablespoons	
Each serving has:			
3.2g carbohydrate	14.1g fat	0.8g fiber	0.4g protein

1 clove garlic, pulverized (use a *mortar* and *pestle*)

Juice of 1 medium lemon

2 TB. avocado oil

Pinch sea salt

Pinch freshly ground black pepper

1. In a mortar; small, nonmetallic bowl; or prep dish, combine garlic, lemon juice, avocado oil, sea salt, and black pepper.

2. Use the pestle or the back of a spoon to mash and thoroughly swirl ingredients together.

3. Allow dressing to rest for 8 to 10 minutes while flavors meld. Taste and adjust seasonings, if necessary.

4. Serve immediately over your favorite salad or alongside crudités.

DEFINITION

A **mortar** is a sturdy bowl, typically made of ceramic or stone, in which hard spices, herbs, or medicines are ground. A **pestle** is a dense, club-shape tool that grinds the materials in the mortar.

Dilly Tofu-Cream Dressing

Creamy herb dressings like this one allow you to enjoy the taste of dairy without the acid-forming ingredients.

Yield:	Prep time:	Serving size:	
2 cups	5 minutes	2 tablespoons	
Each serving has:			
2g carbohydrate	3g fat	0g fiber	7g protein

1 lb. extra-firm tofu, rinsed

2 TB. freshly squeezed lemon juice

1 TB. organic brown rice vinegar

2 tsp. ume plum vinegar

⅓ cup fresh chives, finely chopped

⅓ cup fresh dill, finely chopped

¼ cup water

2 cloves garlic, minced

1 TB. fresh parsley, minced

1 tsp. organic maple syrup

1. In a blender or food processor fitted with a chopping blade, purée extra-firm tofu, lemon juice, brown rice vinegar, ume plum vinegar, chives, dill, water, garlic, parsley, and maple syrup until smooth and creamy.

2. To serve, spoon over salad greens or place in a bowl as a dip for crudités or sea vegetable chips.

ACID ALERT!

While most dairy products are only moderately acid forming, people often lose track of how much dairy they consume. Cheeses, butter, whey, casein, milk and milk solids, cream, and yogurt are prominent ingredients in many processed foods—including salad dressings—and quickly tip your acid/alkaline balance.

Pumpkin Seed Dressing

Earthy-flavored pumpkin seeds add interesting texture and healthy oils, minerals, and fiber to this salad topper.

Yield:	Prep time:	Serving size:	
1 cup	5 minutes	2 to 4 tablespoons	
Each serving has:			
3g carbohydrate	8g fat	3g fiber	6g protein

½ cup roasted pumpkin seeds (pepitas)

2 TB. fresh parsley, minced

3 TB. green onions, chopped

2 tsp. umeboshi paste

½ cup water

1. In a blender or food processor fitted with a chopping blade, process pumpkin seeds, parsley, green onions, umeboshi paste, and water until creamy.

2. Serve over steamed or blanched vegetables, salads, or fish.

PHABULOUS PHACT

Pepitas (from the Spanish *pepita de calabaza*, or "little seed of squash"), or pumpkin seeds, are sold either hulled or unhulled, and are usually salted and roasted. They make a healthy addition to salads and soups, and are a good source of vegetable protein, magnesium, and zinc.

Poppin' Happy Amaranth Salad Dressing

Children love helping make this fun salad dressing with the silly name and nutty flavor.

Yield:	Prep time:	Cook time:	Serving size:
1½ cups	5 minutes	5 minutes	2 tablespoons

Each serving has:			
4.3g carbohydrate	1.9g fat	.6g fiber	1g protein

½ cup *amaranth*	2 TB. tamari soy sauce
1 cup light olive oil	2 cloves garlic, minced

1. In a dry, heavy-bottom skillet over medium to medium-high heat, toast amaranth until it begins to pop. Place a colander over the skillet to catch any escaping amaranth seeds, and continue to pop seeds by swirling the skillet around so seeds don't burn.

2. When half to most of seeds have popped, remove the skillet from heat.

3. In a small bowl, whisk amaranth, olive oil, tamari soy sauce, and garlic together until well combined.

4. Place in a glass jar with a lid, screw on the lid, and refrigerate overnight to allow flavors to meld.

5. Shake well before using, and serve drizzled over your favorite fresh vegetable salad.

DEFINITION

Amaranth is an ancient high-protein crop originating in the Americas that has been shown to reduce cholesterol. It can be used whole, ground into flour for use in baked goods, popped like popcorn, or flaked like oatmeal.

Super Snacks and Dips

In This Chapter

- Planning for snack-time success
- Handy foods to stock up on
- Satisfying snacks to prevent temptation

Don't think that just because you're balancing your diet, you can't indulge in a snack from time to time. On the contrary, it's important to snack and especially *plan* your snacks.

Old habits and constant temptations lurk around every corner, so it's important to have yummy, healthy snacks on hand to avoid falling prey. Veggie sticks and fresh fruit make for perfectly balanced alkaline snacking, but eating plain fruits and vegetables all the time can get boring. Sometimes you'll really crave things like potato chips and cheese dip or homemade cookies. When these old nemeses come haunting, the recipes in this chapter will help keep those unbalanced cravings at bay.

Crisp Nori Chips with Toasted Sesame Oil

Smoky-flavored sesame oil complements nori's natural saltiness and hints of ocean freshness in these chips.

Yield:	Prep time:	Cook time:	Serving size:
60 nori chips	5 minutes	20 minutes	20 nori chips
Each serving has:			
20g carbohydrate	0g fat	trace fiber	20g protein

8 *nori* sheets

1 generous pinch sea salt

1 TB. toasted sesame oil

1. Preheat the oven to 250°F.

2. Lightly brush each nori sheet with a little water, lightly sprinkle with sea salt, and fold in half. Stack folded nori sheets, and cut into 1-inch strips using a sharp knife or pizza cutter.

3. Place nori strips in a single layer on a baking sheet, and bake for 15 to 20 minutes or until dark and crisp.

4. Slide chips onto a wire rack to cool.

5. Lightly brush cooled chips with toasted sesame seed oil, and serve.

DEFINITION

Nori is an edible seaweed used extensively in Japanese cuisine, most notably in fashioning sushi rolls.

pH Pizza Pockets

Zucchini, tomatoes, basil, and oregano echo the familiar flavors of pizza in this sensational sandwich.

Yield:	Prep time:	Cook time:	Serving size:
4 pizza pockets	15 minutes	20 minutes	1 pizza pocket

Each serving has:			
54g carbohydrate	4.5g fat	7.6g fiber	8.5g protein

1 pt. grape or cherry tomatoes, halved

¹/₂ cup green onions, white and green parts, chopped

1 TB. plus ¹/₃ cup water

2 TB. fresh basil, chopped

1 TB. fresh oregano

2 cups buckwheat flour

2 tsp. baking powder

2 tsp. olive oil

1 medium zucchini, cut into ¹/₂-in. slices

1. Preheat the oven to 350°F.

2. In a small saucepan over low heat, simmer grape tomatoes, green onions, and 1 tablespoon water for 5 minutes.

3. Remove from heat, stir in basil and oregano, and set aside to cool.

4. In a medium bowl, combine buckwheat flour and baking powder. Stir in olive oil and remaining ¹/₃ cup water to form a soft dough.

5. Divide dough into 4 balls, and flatten each into a circle on lightly floured parchment paper.

6. Divide tomato mixture among dough circles, and top each with zucchini slices. Fold over dough, and crimp edges to close pocket, creating 4 half-moon shapes.

7. Lifting by the parchment paper, transfer pizza pockets to a baking sheet, and bake for 12 to 15 minutes.

8. Cool for 5 minutes, and serve.

Spiced Roasted Nut Mix

If you love crunchy cereal snack mixes, you'll really enjoy these fragrant nuts spiced with cumin, coriander, chili powder, garlic salt, and ginger.

Yield:	Prep time:	Cook time:	Serving size:
5 cups	5 minutes	20 minutes	1 generous handful
Each serving has:			
3.6g carbohydrate	13.1g fat	1.8g fiber	3.5g protein

1 tsp. ground coriander

$\frac{1}{2}$ tsp. salt

$\frac{1}{2}$ tsp. cumin

$\frac{1}{2}$ tsp. chili powder

$\frac{1}{2}$ tsp. garlic salt

$\frac{1}{4}$ tsp. ground cinnamon

$\frac{1}{4}$ tsp. ground ginger

$\frac{1}{4}$ tsp. cayenne

2 TB. olive oil

$\frac{1}{2}$ cup raw sunflower seeds, shelled

$\frac{1}{2}$ cup raw pumpkin seeds, shelled

1 cup raw almonds, shelled

1 cup raw pecans, shelled

1 TB. coarse sea salt (optional)

1. Preheat the oven to 350°F. Line a baking sheet with aluminum foil or parchment paper.

2. In a small jar with a lid, add coriander, salt, cumin, chili powder, garlic salt, cinnamon, ginger, and cayenne. Add the lid, and shake vigorously for a few seconds to mix spices.

3. In a small nonstick skillet over low heat, heat olive oil. Stir in spices, and toast lightly, stirring constantly, for about 5 minutes. The fragrance will tell you when spices are done.

4. In a medium bowl, toss together sunflower seeds, pumpkin seeds, almonds, pecans, and toasted spices. Evenly spread mixture onto the prepared baking sheet, and bake for 15 minutes, stirring twice at 3- to 5-minute intervals.

5. Remove the baking sheet from the oven, and sprinkle nuts with sea salt (if using). Cool completely.

6. Store in an airtight container for up to 2 weeks.

BALANCE BONUS

Pack a handful of spiced mixed nuts in snack-size zipper-lock plastic bags to keep in the car, your purse, or at your desk. When snack cravings come at high-temptation times of day, you'll be ready!

pH-Style Tortilla Chips

These crisp, earthy, chili powder–enhanced chips are just the thing to complement a variety of yummy pH balance dips.

Yield:	Prep time:	Cook time:	Serving size:
36 to 40 chips	30 minutes	10 minutes	6 to 8 chips
Each serving has:			
29.4g carbohydrate	0.8g fat	4.9g fiber	5.5g protein

2 cups spelt flour	¼ cup olive oil
1 tsp. baking powder	½ to ¾ cup warm water
½ tsp. salt	1 TB. chili powder, or to taste

1. Preheat the oven to 350°F.

2. In a large bowl, stir together spelt flour, baking powder, and salt. Add olive oil and, using your hands, mix oil into dry ingredients until thoroughly incorporated. Add warm water a little at a time, until a sticky ball of dough forms.

3. Form dough into 6 balls, return them to the bowl, cover, and allow to rest for 30 minutes.

4. Using additional spelt flour, lightly dust a pastry board or your countertop, and roll out each dough ball into a $\frac{1}{8}$-inch-thick circle about 6 or 7 inches in diameter.

5. Heat a dry, cast-iron skillet over medium-high heat. Add 1 dough circle to the hot skillet, and cook for about 30 seconds or until bubbles form on the surface. Turn over dough, and cook for about 30 more seconds. Repeat with remaining dough.

6. Cut tortillas into 6 or 8 wedges, and arrange in a single layer on a baking sheet. Sprinkle with chili powder, and bake for 10 minutes or until lightly toasted.

7. Serve chips on their own or with a healthy pH balance dip.

ACID ALERT!

These tortilla crisps won't contribute to an acid imbalance—if eaten in moderation. But to make them a truly alkalizing snack, pair them with an alkalizing dip. You'll feel full sooner and get more nutrition at the same time.

Baba Ghanoush

This Middle Eastern dish boasts a wonderful balance of flavor and texture defined by creamy, smoky eggplant contrasted with bright lemon and garlic. Tahini lends it some body, while the coconut oil makes for an exotic finish.

Yield:	Prep time:	Cook time:	Serving size:
2 cups	5 minutes	45 minutes	$\frac{1}{4}$ cup

Each serving has:			
4.1g carbohydrate	7.1g fat	2g fiber	0.7g protein

1 large eggplant	2 cloves garlic, crushed and peeled
$\frac{1}{4}$ cup virgin coconut oil	$\frac{1}{4}$ cup tahini
Salt	Extra-virgin olive oil (optional)
Coarsely ground black pepper	
3 TB. freshly squeezed lemon juice	

1. Preheat the oven to 350°F.

2. Cut eggplant in half lengthwise. Without piercing the skin, score the cut surfaces $1/2$ inch deep in a diamond pattern from edge to edge. Brush each scored surface with 1 tablespoon virgin coconut oil, and sprinkle liberally with salt and black pepper.

3. Place cut side down on a baking sheet, and roast for 45 minutes or until flesh is very soft. Remove from oven, and set aside to cool.

4. With a large spoon, scoop out eggplant flesh and add to a food processor fitted with a chopping blade. Add lemon juice, garlic, and tahini, and purée.

5. Add remaining coconut oil and blend again. Taste for salt and pepper, and adjust seasoning if necessary.

6. Serve *baba ganoush* in a large dip bowl, drizzled with extra-virgin olive oil (if using), alongside a variety of fresh-cut vegetables and pita chips.

DEFINITION

Baba ganoush is a traditional Middle Eastern eggplant dish typically served with warm pita bread and an assortment of crudités.

Wholly Guacamole

Brightened by fresh cilantro, fresh lemon juice, and sweet red onion, this creamy, cool Mexican-flavored dip goes well with chips and raw veggies sticks, or as topping for grilled whitefish or veggie burgers.

Yield:	Prep time:	Serving size:
3½ cups	10 minutes, plus 30 minutes chill time	½ cup

Each serving has:			
6.5g carbohydrate	12.5g fat	4.3g fiber	1.4g protein

2 ripe avocados, peeled and pitted

2 TB. extra-virgin olive oil

1 TB. freshly squeezed lime juice

¼ tsp. sea salt

2 small tomatoes, diced

¼ cup fresh cilantro, chopped

¼ cup red onion, finely chopped

1 tsp. hot pepper sauce

1. In a medium nonmetallic bowl, and using a fork, mash together avocados, extra-virgin olive oil, lime juice, and sea salt until well combined.

2. Stir in tomatoes, cilantro, red onion, and hot pepper sauce.

3. Cover and refrigerate for 30 minutes.

4. Stir and serve.

ACID ALERT!

Some of the most acidifying foods are artificial sweeteners, black olives, cheese, coffee, corn, wheat flour, and refined sugar. While you should not strive to completely eliminate all acid-forming foods from your diet, in order to maintain a good balance, you must be aware of how much and how often you consume them.

Garlicky Cucumber Dip

Garlic lovers will rejoice over this dip made with cooling cucumbers, sweet mint, and a distinct garlic bite.

Yield:	Prep time:	Serving size:	
2 cups	5 minutes	¼ cup	
Each serving has:			
32.4g carbohydrate	9.1g fat	6.1g fiber	6.8g protein

1 (12-oz.) pkg. soft tofu

3 cloves garlic, mashed and minced

1 handful fresh mint leaves, chopped

½ medium cucumber, diced

Freshly squeezed lemon juice

1. In a food processor fitted with a chopping blade, blend together tofu, garlic, and mint leaves until smooth.

2. Spoon mixture into a medium nonmetallic bowl, add cucumber, and stir well.

3. Stir in lemon juice, 1 teaspoon at a time, to taste.

4. Serve immediately, or cover and refrigerate until ready to serve. Flavors will intensify with time.

PHABULOUS PHACT

You can increase garlic's health benefits by letting it sit for a few minutes after you've mashed or chopped it. Chopping or crushing garlic stimulates a process that converts the phytonutrient alliin into allicin, the latter of which many of garlic's health benefits have been attributed to. Letting crushed garlic sit for 10 minutes before cooking or combining it with other foods preserves the full spectrum of its healthful properties.

Hearty Spinach Dip

This dip is has an earthly taste reminiscent of humus, but with the added benefit of refreshing and alkalizing spinach.

Yield:	Prep time:	Serving size:	
3 cups	5 minutes	⅓ cup	
Each serving has:			
41.2g carbohydrate	11.1g fat	14.8g fiber	14g protein

1 ripe avocado, peeled and pitted

Juice of ½ medium lemon

1 (8-oz.) can chickpeas, rinsed and drained

1 (10-oz.) pkg. chopped frozen spinach, thawed and squeezed dry

1. In a food processor fitted with a chopping blade, process avocado, lemon juice, and chickpeas until smooth.

2. Add spinach, and process again until evenly incorporated.

3. Scoop into a nonmetallic bowl and serve immediately, or cover and refrigerate until ready to serve.

BALANCE BONUS

Be sure to include plenty of chlorophyll-rich leafy greens in your diet. They cleanse your blood and alkalize you, too.

Avocado Cream Sauce

Lemon zest and freshly squeezed lemon juice brighten up the creaminess of this easy avocado sauce.

Yield:	Prep time:	Serving size:	
1 cup	5 minutes	¼ cup	
Each serving has:			
10.3g carbohydrate	17.6g fat	8.1g fiber	2.6g protein

2 small to medium ripe Hass avocados, peeled and seeded	4 TB. freshly squeezed lemon juice
1 tsp. fresh lemon zest	

1. In a blender, purée Hass avocados, lemon zest, and lemon juice until smooth and creamy, adding more lemon juice as desired.

2. Pour into a small glass bowl, cover with plastic wrap to prevent browning, and refrigerate until ready to serve.

BALANCE BONUS

This sauce also is delicious served as a dip with fresh vegetables, as a spread on veggie burgers, and even as a salad dressing.

Hearty Entrées

In This Chapter

- Perfect poultry dishes
- Super-easy slow cooker recipes
- Sensational seafood suppers

Vegetables and fruits, juices and smoothies are part of the pH balance diet, but by now you should be realizing they're not *all* you'll be eating as you work to bring your body's pH in balance.

In this chapter, I share some recipes for mouthwatering main dishes. From tasty turkey meatballs, to comforting shepherd's pie, to satisfying seafood lasagna, and much more, you'll love the balancing entrées in this chapter.

Turkey Meatballs in Chunky Garden Vegetable Sauce

Served in a chunky vegetable sauce of tomatoes, squash, and potatoes, these garlic- and cilantro-seasoned meatballs are delicious.

Yield:	Prep time:	Cook time:	Serving size:
20 meatballs and 2 quarts sauce	10 minutes	45 minutes	5 meatballs and 2 cups sauce

Each serving has:			
24g carbohydrate	3.9g fat	4.4g fiber	34.2g protein

1 (14-oz.) can diced tomatoes

1 clove garlic, finely sliced

1 medium yellow onion, roughly chopped

1 large celery rib, thinly sliced

1 large carrot, trimmed and sliced

1 medium russet or your choice potato, peeled and cubed

1 large leek, white and tender green parts, cleaned well and cut into 1-in. slices

1 large yellow crook-neck squash, cut into $\frac{1}{2}$-in. slices

$1\frac{1}{3}$ cups water

1 lb. ground turkey

1 medium yellow onion, finely chopped

1 clove garlic, mashed and minced

1 handful fresh cilantro, minced

$\frac{1}{2}$ tsp. organic vegetable bouillon paste

1. Preheat the oven to 350°F.

2. In a large saucepan or Dutch oven over medium-high heat, combine tomatoes, sliced garlic, roughly chopped yellow onion, celery, carrot, potato, leek, yellow crook-neck squash, and water. Bring to a boil, reduce heat to medium-low, and simmer, stirring occasionally, for 30 minutes.

3. Meanwhile, in a large bowl and using your hands, knead together ground turkey, finely chopped yellow onion, minced garlic, cilantro, and vegetable bouillon paste.

4. Form turkey mixture into 20 small meatballs, place them on a baking sheet, and bake for 15 minutes.

5. Meanwhile, using an immersion blender, carefully purée a portion of vegetable sauce in the saucepan so it thickens but some vegetable chunks remain.

6. Add meatballs to sauce, stir, and simmer for a few more minutes so meatballs absorb sauce's flavors.

7. Serve hot, accompanied by a crisp green salad and a squeeze of lemon.

ACID ALERT!

Eating properly goes a long way toward fighting acidosis, but water is important, too. Besides the water you drink and use in tea, consider how much water goes into making your foods—especially soups and sauces. Using spring water helps ensure your water has an alkaline or neutral pH.

Shepherd's Pie

This vegetarian shepherd's pie is so full of garden-fresh vegetables, you'll never miss the meat.

Yield:	Prep time:	Cook time:	Serving size:
1 13×9×2-inch casserole	15 minutes	45 minutes	$\frac{1}{4}$ of casserole

Each serving has:			
130.6g carbohydrate	1.4g fat	29.2g fiber	31g protein

4 medium sweet potatoes, peeled and cubed

Dash *tamari*

2 TB. olive oil

1 clove garlic, crushed and minced

1 medium yellow onion, halved and sliced

2 medium celery ribs, chopped

1 small butternut squash, peeled, seeded, and diced

2 cups organic vegetable stock

1 (15-oz.) can organic kidney beans, rinsed and drained

1 large red or yellow bell pepper, ribs and seeds removed, and chopped

4 medium tomatoes, trimmed and halved

2 medium zucchini, sliced

1 medium head broccoli, chopped

3 medium carrots, sliced

2 TB. fresh parsley, chopped

1 tsp. arrowroot

1. Preheat the oven to 400°F.

2. Place sweet potatoes in a steamer, set over medium-high heat, and steam for 15 minutes or until soft.

3. Transfer potatoes to a food processor fitted with a chopping blade, add tamari, and process until smooth. Set aside.

4. In a large saucepan over medium heat, heat olive oil. Add garlic, yellow onion, and celery, and sauté for about 5 minutes.

5. Add butternut squash, and sauté for about 5 more minutes.

6. Stir in vegetable stock, and bring to a boil. Reduce heat to low, and simmer for about 10 minutes.

7. Stir in kidney beans, red bell pepper, tomatoes, zucchini, broccoli, carrots, and parsley, and cook for about 10 minutes or until butternut squash is tender.

8. Remove from heat, stir in arrowroot, and transfer vegetables to a 13×9×2-inch casserole dish.

9. Top with puréed sweet potatoes, and bake for 15 to 20 minutes or until casserole is set. Cool for 5 minutes before serving.

> **DEFINITION**
>
> **Tamari** is a naturally fermented premium soy sauce made with extremely little wheat or none at all.

Steamy Salmon Lasagna

Savoy cabbage replaces pasta in this lasagna and contributes a natural sweetness to this dish that's sure to become a family favorite.

Yield:	Prep time:	Cook time:	Serving size:
1 13×9×2-inch casserole	15 minutes	45 minutes	¼ of casserole

Each serving has:			
21.8g carbohydrate	4.7g fat	8.6g fiber	25.3g protein

1 large head savoy cabbage	1 tsp. tamari
2 tsp. sesame oil	1 (1-lb.) salmon fillet
¼ cup water	8 medium green onions, white and green parts, chopped
Zest of 1 medium lemon	
2 tsp. brown rice vinegar	

1. Bring a large pot of water to a boil over medium-high heat.

2. Discard tough outer leaves from head of savoy cabbage. Carefully remove 5 leaves and, using a sharp knife, cut out and discard toughest part of central vein in each leaf. Drop leaves into boiling water, and blanch for 2 minutes. Drain and rinse under cold running water.

3. Using the knife, core and shred remaining cabbage.

4. In a large saucepan over medium heat, bring sesame oil and water to a boil. Add shredded cabbage, and cook for 2 minutes or until cabbage has wilted. Remove from heat.

5. Stir in lemon zest, brown rice vinegar, and tamari, and set aside.

6. Using a very sharp knife, slice salmon against the grain into $\frac{1}{8}$-inch slices.

7. To assemble, stack 2 blanched cabbage leaves in the middle of a long sheet of waxed paper, and top with $\frac{1}{3}$ of salmon. Spoon $\frac{1}{3}$ of shredded cabbage onto salmon, and top with another blanched cabbage leaf. Continue layering salmon, shredded cabbage, and cabbage leaf until all of salmon and cabbage has been used.

8. Pull up the sides of the waxed paper, and firmly enclose lasagna. Firmly tuck waxed paper package into a bamboo steamer, set over medium-high heat, and steam for 10 minutes. Remove from heat.

9. Carefully remove package from the steamer, cut lasagna into 4 portions, garnish with green onions, and serve hot.

> **PHABULOUS PHACT**
>
> Besides being an alkalizing food, cabbage offers many health benefits. It's high in free radical–fighting antioxidants and anti-inflammatory polyphenols, and it's has been shown to aid in stomach ulcer and cancer prevention. Cabbage also is a good source of an amino acid called l-glutamine that's instrumental in restoring the lining of the intestines.

Slow-Cooker Cassoulet

Slow cooking enables the garlic, rosemary, and thyme to infuse their flavor into the tender beans. Store leftovers in the refrigerator, and enjoy the deepening flavors for days to come!

Yield:	Prep time:	Cook time:	Serving size:
3 quarts	15 minutes	6 to 8 hours	2 cups

Each serving has:			
48.2g carbohydrate	1.3g fat	15.5g fiber	16g protein

1 cup dried navy beans, rinsed and sorted	2 cloves garlic, minced
1 cup dried pinto beans, rinsed and sorted	2 sprigs fresh rosemary
	2 sprigs fresh thyme
1 medium yellow onion, chopped	1 tsp. fennel seed
1 large leek, white and tender green parts, split vertically and cut into ½-in. slices	4 roma tomatoes, chopped
	2 TB. fresh parsley, chopped
	6 cups water

1. In a 5- to 7-quart slow cooker, add navy beans, pinto beans, yellow onion, leek, garlic, rosemary, thyme, fennel seed, roma tomatoes, and parsley.

2. Pour in water, stir once to evenly distribute ingredients, cover, and cook on high for 6 to 8 hours or until beans are soft and creamy.

3. Serve over freshly cooked brown rice.

BALANCE BONUS

Cassoulet is a rich, slow-cooked one-pot meal featuring creamy beans that originated in southern France. Traditional cassoulets are made with *haricots blanc* (white beans), but you can substitute other dried beans in this recipe and still get delicious results.

Slow-Cooked Red Lentil Curry

Cilantro, lime, turmeric, cumin, and ginger transform sweet and nutty red lentils into an Indian curry bursting with exotic flavors.

Yield:	Prep time:	Cook time:	Serving size:
1½ quarts	15 minutes	6 to 8 hours	1 cup

Each serving has:			
50.4g carbohydrate	4.5g fat	20.4g fiber	16.6g protein

2 medium tomatoes, diced

2 medium green onions, white and green parts, sliced

2 TB. fresh cilantro, chopped

1 TB. freshly squeezed lime juice

1 TB. olive oil

1 medium yellow onion, chopped

1 clove garlic, minced

1 tsp. ground cumin

½ tsp. turmeric

½ tsp. ground ginger

1 cup split red lentils, gently rinsed and sorted

2 medium carrots, trimmed and sliced

1 medium sweet potato, peeled and cut into 1-in. cubes

½ (6-oz.) box frozen peas

3 cups water

1. In a nonmetallic bowl, combine tomatoes, green onions, cilantro, lime juice, and olive oil. Stir well, cover, and refrigerate.

2. In a 5- to 7-quart slow cooker, add yellow onion, garlic, cumin, turmeric, ginger, split red lentils, carrots, sweet potato, and frozen peas.

3. Pour in water, stir once to evenly distribute ingredients, cover, and cook on high for 6 to 8 hours.

4. Serve over freshly cooked brown rice accompanied by the chilled tomato relish.

PHABULOUS PHACT

Most herbs and spices are full of powerful antioxidants, vitamins, and minerals that help your body stay healthfully alkaline. Experiment with different spices and herbs, and enjoy improved health!

Asian Tempeh Cutlet Salad

Ginger-spiced tempeh is accompanied by the freshness of mixed baby greens, mung bean sprouts, and daikon radish in this Asian-inspired dinner salad.

Yield:	Prep time:	Cook time:	Serving size:
4 tempeh dinner salads	5 minutes	12 minutes	1 salad

Each serving has:			
18.8g carbohydrate	7.6g fat	4.5g fiber	16.1g protein

1 (8-oz.) pkg. *tempeh*	4 cups mixed baby greens
12 (¼-in.) slices fresh ginger	1 cup raw mung bean sprouts
1 tsp. sesame oil	1 (2-in.) piece *daikon* radish,
¼ cup water	julienned
Dash tamari	

1. Place tempeh in a bamboo steamer, cover with ginger slices, set over medium-high heat, and steam for 10 minutes.

2. Remove tempeh, discard ginger, and slice tempeh into ½-inch strips.

3. In a medium skillet over medium-high heat, heat sesame oil and water. Add tempeh, cut side down, and cook for 1 minute. Turn over tempeh, sprinkle with tamari, and cook for 1 more minute.

4. Arrange mixed baby greens, mung bean sprouts, and daikon radish in a mound on 4 dinner plates, top with tempeh, drizzle with sauce from the skillet, and serve immediately.

DEFINITION

Tempeh is a meaty Indonesian soy product that easily takes on the flavors of foods it's cooked with. **Daikon,** meaning "large root," is the Japanese name for a large—up to 14 inches long and 4 inches in diameter—mildly flavored white radish commonly used in Asian cuisine. In the Europe and continental Asia, it's commonly called *mooli*.

Lemony Chicken Burgers

Lemon is the bright highlight of these light and yummy chicken burgers.

Yield:	Prep time:	Cook time:	Serving size:
4 burgers	5 minutes	20 minutes	1 burger

Each serving has:			
2.5g carbohydrate	15.4g fat	trace fiber	33.2g protein

1 TB. olive oil

1 small white or yellow onion, chopped

1 small leek, white and tender green parts, split in half lengthwise and sliced in $\frac{1}{2}$-in. pieces

1 clove garlic, crushed and minced

1 lb. ground chicken

$\frac{1}{2}$ tsp. organic vegetable bouillon paste

1 TB. freshly squeezed lemon juice

Zest of 1 medium lemon

1. Preheat the oven to 400°F. Line a baking sheet with parchment paper.

2. In a medium skillet over medium heat, heat olive oil. Add white onion, leek, and garlic, and *sweat* for a few minutes. Do not allow to brown. Set aside until cool enough to handle.

3. In a medium bowl, and using your hands, knead together onion mixture, chicken, vegetable bouillon paste, lemon juice, and lemon zest.

4. Form mixture into 4 balls, place on the prepared baking sheet, and flatten to form patties.

5. Bake for 10 minutes. Flip over patties, and bake for 5 more minutes.

6. Serve hot or cold accompanied by a large crisp salad and vinaigrette of choice.

> **DEFINITION**
>
> To **sweat** vegetables means to cook them over low heat in a small amount of fat, stirring often, while allowing them to soften and release moisture but not brown.

Whitefish with Braised Fennel

Fragrant anise and fennel define this easy entrée that's done in minutes.

Yield:	Prep time:	Cook time:	Serving size:
4 fillets	5 minutes	25 minutes	1 fillet
Each serving has:			
9.8g carbohydrate	0.2g fat	3.9 fiber	22.1g protein

2 medium blubs fennel, finely sliced	4 (4-oz.) fresh cod, haddock, flounder, or other whitefish fillets
2 star anise	
1 cup boiling water	1 medium lemon, sliced crosswise into wagon wheels

1. Preheat the oven to 350°F.

2. In a 13×9×2-inch ovenproof baking dish, add fennel, star anise, and boiling water. Bake for 15 minutes.

3. Remove baking dish from the oven. Place whitefish fillets on fennel, top with lemon slices, and bake for 10 more minutes or until fish is opaque and easily flakes with a fork.

4. Serve immediately.

> **PHABULOUS PHACT**
>
> Star anise is an Asian spice commonly used by herbalists and in traditional medicine to reduce intestinal gas, aid digestion, and act as a powerful diuretic. It's also a major ingredient in some antiviral pharmaceuticals such as the flu medication Tamiflu.

Simply Salmon for One

The simple, clean, ocean flavor of salmon with steamed fresh carrots and broccoli contrasts nicely with light and crispy salad greens.

Yield:	Prep time:	Cook time:	Serving size:
1 salmon fillet	5 minutes	20 minutes	1 salmon fillet

Each serving has:			
9.8g carbohydrate	0.2g fat	3.9g fiber	22.1g protein

1 (6-oz.) salmon fillet	2 cups salad greens
2 medium carrots, cut into carrot sticks	2 to 4 lemon and lime wedges
1 small head broccoli, cut into florets	

1. Preheat the oven to 350°F. Line a baking sheet with parchment paper.

2. Place salmon on the prepared baking sheet, and bake for 20 minutes or until firm and opaque.

3. Meanwhile, place carrots and broccoli florets in a bamboo steamer, set over medium-high heat, and steam for 5 or 6 minutes or until tender-crisp.

4. Serve salmon hot along with steamed carrots and broccoli, salad greens, and lemon and lime wedges, squeezing lemon and lime over fish, vegetables, and/or salad greens as you like.

BALANCE BONUS

If you live alone, it's often uninspiring to cook for yourself, and it becomes tempting to eat unhealthy convenience foods. To make things easier on yourself, think in terms of simple meals like this one. The salmon bakes while you steam the broccoli and carrots—making a quick, complete, filling meal. Or create something more extravagant on the weekend and store portions in the refrigerator or freezer for easy meals another day.

Asian Poached Chicken for One

Ginger, cilantro, and miso deliver distinctive Asian flavor in this quick and tasty dish.

Yield:	Prep time:	Cook time:	Serving size:
1 chicken breast	5 minutes	15 minutes	1 chicken breast
Each serving has:			
17.2g carbohydrate	2g fat	5.4g fiber	60.4g protein

1 (6 to 8-oz.) free-range chicken breast

1¼ cups organic vegetable stock

1 TB. organic miso paste

1 (1-in.) piece fresh ginger

2 cloves garlic, minced

3 TB. fresh cilantro, chopped

2 baby bok choy, trimmed and roughly chopped

½ medium red bell pepper, ribs and seeds removed, and finely sliced

1 handful fresh mung, aduki, lentil, or your choice bean sprouts

1. Preheat the oven to 400°F.

2. Place chicken breast in the center of a 9×9-inch baking pan. Set aside.

3. In a small saucepan over medium heat, bring vegetable stock to a boil. Remove from heat, and stir in miso paste, ginger, garlic, and 2 tablespoons cilantro.

4. Pour stock mixture over chicken, cover the pan with aluminum foil, and bake for 10 minutes.

5. Arrange baby bok choy on a plate, and top with chicken, red bell pepper slices, and mung bean sprouts. Spoon some hot stock over all, garnish with remaining 1 tablespoon cilantro, and serve immediately.

PHABULOUS PHACT

According to a study published in the June 2004 issue of the *Journal of Agriculture and Food Chemistry*, cilantro contains dodecenal, a powerful antibacterial compound that's twice as effective as gentamicin at killing salmonella. Salmonella, which often occurs in chicken, is a common and sometimes deadly cause of food-borne illness, so cilantro makes a perfect herb choice for chicken dishes.

Soups and Stews

In This Chapter

- Super soups and stocks
- Soups for every meal
- Hearty and nourishing soups and stews

Soups and stews can easily form the basis of a pH balance diet and provide dense nutrition while demanding little in the way of preparation and attention. Only the wholesome produce available to you and your imagination limit the variety of flavor profiles you can achieve in your soup bowl.

I encourage you to try to include a serving of soup at every meal. Beyond just lunch and dinner, have, for instance, some warm, mineral-rich miso soup for breakfast. And raw blended or chilled soups make for quick and easy nutritious snacks.

You can start a batch of soup in your slow cooker in the morning, and let your slow cooker do all the work. At dinnertime, you'll have a perfectly cooked soup ready for dinner. Or start your slow cooker the night before, and you'll have lunch ready to pack before you leave for work the next morning!

Hippocrates Soup

This recipe, developed by Dr. Max Gerson for his healing therapy, provides a nice balance of earthly, warm vegetable flavors. It's a bowl full of autumn harvest goodness.

Yield:	Prep time:	Cook time:	Serving size:
4 quarts	5 minutes	2 hours	1 cup

Each serving has:			
11.2g carbohydrate	0.2g fat	2.4g fiber	1.5g protein

1 medium celery root or 4 celery ribs	1½ lb. tomatoes
1 medium parsnip	2 medium onions
1 clove garlic	1 lb. your choice potatoes
2 small leeks	1 small bunch fresh parsley

1. Wash and scrub vegetables well, leave the skins on, and chop into coarse chunks.

2. In a 5-quart stainless-steel pot over medium heat, combine celery root, parsnip, garlic, leeks, tomatoes, onions potatoes, and parsley, along with just enough water to cover vegetables. Simmer slowly for 2 hours.

3. Using a food mill or a kitchen sieve, process soup in small batches until only vegetable fibers and peelings remain in the mill.

4. Serve puréed soup warm. Store leftover soup covered in the refrigerator for up to 2 days, and reheat individual servings when ready to eat.

BALANCE BONUS

Gerson Therapy–based recipes are especially good at balancing pH and are highly therapeutic on a cellular level. Because of their high potassium content, you'll notice reduced fluid retention, which allows your cells to cleanse and take in nutrients at an optimal level. Dr. Gerson prescribes 1 cup Hippocrates Soup for his patients at every meal. This recipe produces a fairly thick soup, but you can adjust the amount of water you use to suit your tastes and desired consistency.

Tomato Soup with Lemon and Garlic

The relative acidity of the tomatoes in this soup is balanced by the alkalizing effect of the zesty lemon and the high potassium content of the Hippocrates Soup.

Yield:	Prep time:	Cook time:	Serving size:
4 cups	5 minutes	1 hour	1 cup

Each serving has:			
14.8g carbohydrate	0.45g fat	3.3g fiber	2.3g protein

3 large tomatoes, diced

1 clove garlic, minced

1 bay leaf

Juice of ½ medium lemon

2 medium yellow onions, diced

1 tsp. brown sugar

½ cup Hippocrates Soup (recipe earlier in this chapter)

1 tsp. rolled oats

1. In a medium saucepan over medium heat, combine tomatoes, garlic, bay leaf, lemon juice, yellow onions, brown sugar, and Hippocrates Soup. Bring to a boil, reduce heat to medium-low, and simmer for 1 hour.

2. Remove bay leaf and, using an immersion blender, purée soup in the pan.

3. Add rolled oats, and cook for 5 more minutes.

4. Serve immediately.

PHABULOUS PHACT

Garlic has many proven health benefits, including antibacterial properties and the ability to lower cholesterol. Consuming fresh garlic may reduce the blood's ability to clot, however, so anyone with a bleeding disorder should be careful to not overconsume garlic. For the same reason, garlic in supplement form is usually not recommended for women who are pregnant or breast-feeding.

Minted Tomato Soup

The fresh taste of mint and the bright tang of yogurt make this a treat either hot or chilled.

Yield:	Prep time:	Cook time:	Serving size:
6 cups	5 minutes	30 minutes	1½ cups

Each serving has:			
27.7g carbohydrate	1.5g fat	6.2g fiber	6.6g protein

6 medium roma tomatoes, chopped

5 medium green onions, white and green parts, sliced

2 small apples of your choice, cored and sliced

5 TB. cider vinegar

1 tsp. brown sugar

Juice of 2 large lemons

1 cup plain yogurt

6 sprigs fresh mint, chopped

1. In a medium stainless-steel saucepan over medium heat, combine roma tomatoes, green onions, apples, cider vinegar, and brown sugar. Bring to a boil, reduce heat to low, and simmer for 30 minutes.

2. Remove from heat and, using an immersion blender, purée soup in the pan.

3. Stir in lemon juice and yogurt until well combined.

4. Immediately before serving, stir in ½ of mint, and garnish individual bowls with remaining chopped mint.

PHABULOUS PHACT

Mint is well known as a flavoring agent and as a mouth and breath freshener, but it also has remarkable medicinal properties. Mint is an excellent digestion aid, can relieve nausea and headaches, relieves coughs and soothes the throat, and has even shown some benefit in studies of cancer therapies.

Dashi

Dashi is the quintessential Japanese soup stock that provides a depth of smoky, salty, sea-flavored essence and forms the dried fish base of many Asian dishes.

Yield:	Prep time:	Cook time:	Serving size:
1 quart	1 minute	5 minutes	1 cup

Each serving has:			
1.1g carbohydrate	0g fat	1.1g fiber	4.7g protein

1 (4-in.-square) piece kombu	2 medium green onions, white
4 cups water	and green parts, finely sliced
1 oz. dried *bonito flakes*	

1. In a medium saucepan over medium heat, combine kombu and water. Bring to a simmer.

2. Remove kombu from the pan so stock won't foam.

3. Turn off heat, and stir in bonito flakes. When bonito flakes have sunk to the bottom of the pan, strain through a colander and reserve broth.

4. Sprinkle broth with green onions, and serve warm as a nourishing broth, or use as a base for other soups and dishes.

DEFINITION

Bonito flakes are preserved skipjack tuna fish fillet that's been steamed, dried, and shaved into flakes for use as a salty flavored seasoning.

Mineral-Rich Miso Soup

With a vegetable or two from your refrigerator and a little miso paste, the flavor possibilities for miso soup are nearly infinite. Consider adding cabbage, carrot, onion, peas, radish, or kale for variety.

Yield:	Prep time:	Cook time:	Serving size:
1 quart	15 minutes	15 minutes	1 cup

Each serving has:			
15.7g carbohydrate	0.1g fat	2.4g fiber	1.6g protein

1 (4-in.-square) piece kombu

3 dried shiitake mushrooms

4 cups water

2 TB. natural soy sauce

4 TB. white miso paste

6 oz. firm tofu, cut into bite-size cubes

2 medium green onions, white and green parts, sliced

1. Briefly rinse kombu under running water, and blot excess moisture with a clean, damp cloth.

2. In a medium saucepan, combine kombu, shiitake mushrooms, and water, and set aside to soak for 15 minutes.

3. Remove shiitake mushrooms from water, and cut off and discard woody stems. Thinly slice mushroom caps and return to the saucepan. Set over medium heat and bring to a simmer, but do not boil. Simmer for 15 minutes.

4. Using a slotted spoon, remove kombu and shiitake from broth (optional). Stir in soy sauce.

5. Remove the pan from heat, and add white miso paste, stirring until completely dissolved. Stir in tofu, sprinkle soup with green onions, and serve.

BALANCE BONUS

Making and keeping homemade stocks on hand will elevate your meals to gourmet levels. When you make a large pot of soup stock, freeze some in an ice-cube tray, and store the cubes in zipper-lock plastic freezer bags for quick, easy additions to soups or grain and bean dishes.

Spicy Thai Soup with Coconut Milk

The flavor profile of this soup is both balanced and complex, with the cooling qualities of cucumber, mint, and coconut milk providing the perfect balance to the jalapeño's heat.

Yield:	Prep time:	Cook time:	Serving size:
8 cups	10 minutes	40 minutes	2 cups

Each serving has:			
168.4g carbohydrate	25.4g fat	6.7g fiber	22.9g protein

½ cup cucumber, diced

1 medium jalapeño, halved, seeded, and finely sliced

½ cup fresh mint, roughly chopped

1 cup fresh mung bean sprouts, rinsed and drained

½ cup fresh cilantro leaves, roughly chopped

½ lb. (8 oz.) firm tofu, cubed

4 cups cooked medium-grain rice

1 medium yellow onion, chopped

5 cloves garlic, minced

2 stalks lemongrass, trimmed to 1-in. pieces

1 (2-in.) piece fresh ginger, sliced

2 or 3 red chile peppers, chopped

1 tsp. ground cumin

1 TB. ground coriander

½ tsp. turmeric

2 tsp. brown rice syrup

2 TB. coconut oil

5 cups water

¼ cup freshly squeezed lime juice

1 (14-oz.) can coconut milk

1 tsp. sea salt

1 medium lime, quartered (optional)

1. In a large bowl, lightly combine cucumber, jalapeño, mint, mung bean sprouts, cilantro, and tofu. Set aside.

2. Evenly divide medium-grain rice among 4 large soup bowls, and set aside.

3. In a food processor fitted with a chopping blade, process yellow onion, garlic, lemongrass, ginger, red chile peppers, cumin, coriander, turmeric, and brown rice syrup until paste forms.

4. In a heavy-bottomed Dutch oven, heat coconut oil, but don't allow to smoke. Stirring constantly, pour onion mixture into hot oil, and sauté for about 5 to 7 minutes.

5. Stir in water, lime juice, coconut milk, and sea salt, and bring to a boil. Reduce heat to low, and simmer for about 30 more minutes.

6. Strain soup through a colander, reserving soup and discarding solids.

7. Rinse the pot to remove any solids, and return soup to the pot. Set over low heat until ready to serve.

8. Ladle hot soup over each bowl of prepared rice, mound equal amounts of vegetable/tofu mixture in center of each bowl, garnish with 1 fresh lime wedge each (if using), and serve immediately.

BALANCE BONUS

This exotic soup is simple to prepare and takes less than an hour to put together. Most of your energy will be spent in basic prep, though, so assemble your ingredients first and then get started.

Vegetarian Butternut Squash Soup

This creamy butternut squash soup is actually a very mild coconut milk curry. Let the intoxicating flavors and aromas of warm coconut, ginger, turmeric, cumin, and cilantro transport you to the Middle East for dinner tonight!

Yield:	Prep time:	Cook time:	Serving size:
12 cups	10 minutes	30 minutes	1½ cups
Each serving has:			
18.9g carbohydrate	16.6g fat	3.8g fiber	6.4g protein

2 TB. coconut oil	2 tsp. ground cumin
1 large yellow onion, chopped	1 medium butternut squash, peeled, seeded, and cut into ½-in. cubes (about 6 cups)
1 (1-in.) piece fresh ginger, peeled and minced	
6 cloves garlic, crushed and minced	1 (14-oz.) can coconut milk
	Salt
6 cups organic vegetable broth	Freshly ground black pepper
2 tsp. turmeric	¼ cup fresh cilantro, chopped

1. In a medium stockpot over medium heat, heat coconut oil. Add yellow onion, and sauté for 3 to 5 minutes or until translucent. Do not brown onion.

2. Add ginger and garlic, and sauté for 1 or 2 more minutes.

3. Add vegetable broth, turmeric, cumin, and butternut squash; stir to combine; increase heat to high; and bring to a boil. Reduce heat to low and cook, uncovered, for about 10 minutes or until squash is tender.

4. Stir in coconut milk.

5. In a blender, or using an immersion blender, purée soup until completely smooth.

6. Season with salt and fresh black pepper, stir in cilantro, reheat soup if necessary, and serve hot.

Variation: Cool soup in the refrigerator, blend in the flesh of 1 ripe avocado, and serve chilled.

BALANCE BONUS

When cleaning winter squash, save the seeds and toast them in the oven to make a healthy snack or garnish for soups and salads. Squash seeds are an excellent source of hearth-healthy magnesium and fiber.

Sweet Potato, Chipotle, and Kidney Bean Chili

In this vegetarian chili, the smoky heat of chipotle pepper perfectly complements the sweetness of coriander and sweet potatoes.

Yield:	Prep time:	Cook time:	Serving size:
6 cups	10 minutes	60 minutes	1½ cups
Each serving has:			
113.5g carbohydrate	5.6g fat	23.9g fiber	25.1g protein

1 TB. olive oil

1 medium yellow onion, chopped

1 medium red bell pepper, ribs and seeds removed, and chopped

1 large clove garlic, minced

1 TB. chili powder

1 tsp. ground cumin

1 tsp. ground coriander seeds

1½ lb. sweet potatoes, peeled and cubed

2 medium tomatoes, diced

2 cups cooked kidney beans

1½ cups water

1 tsp. Celtic sea salt

1 canned *chipotle pepper*, diced (about 1 TB.)

1. In a large skillet over medium heat, heat olive oil. Add yellow onion, red bell pepper, and garlic. Cover and sweat vegetables for 3 or 4 minutes or until softened but not browned.

2. Quickly add chili powder, cumin, coriander, and sweet potatoes, and stir well to coat.

3. Transfer to a large saucepan, and set over medium heat. Add tomatoes, kidney beans, water, and Celtic sea salt, and bring to a boil. Reduce heat to low, and simmer for 45 minutes or until potatoes are very tender. Or finish in a slow cooker on low for 8 to 10 hours or on high for 6 to 8 hours.

4. Stir in chipotle pepper, and serve immediately.

> **DEFINITION**
>
> A **chipotle pepper** is a ripe, smoked jalapeño. Chipotles are an important spice in Mexican cuisine and provide medium to high heat and a complex, smoky flavor.

Zippy Lentil Soup

The earthiness provided by the lentils and braised fresh vegetables in this soup contrasts nicely with the powerful zing provided by the tomatoes with green chiles and apple cider vinegar.

Yield:	Prep time:	Cook time:	Serving size:
3 quarts	20 minutes	6 to 8 hours	2 cups
Each serving has:			
32g carbohydrate	1g fat	11g fiber	10g protein

1 cup dried lentils, rinsed and sorted

$\frac{1}{3}$ cup pearled barley

2 large carrots, medium diced

$1\frac{1}{2}$ medium celery ribs, diced

1 medium yellow onion, chopped

2 cloves garlic, minced

$\frac{1}{2}$ tsp. dried basil

$\frac{1}{2}$ tsp. dried oregano

$\frac{1}{4}$ tsp. dried thyme

1 bay leaf

$3\frac{1}{2}$ cups water

$3\frac{1}{2}$ cups chicken or vegetable stock

1 (14.5-oz.) can diced tomatoes with green chiles

$\frac{1}{4}$ cup fresh parsley, chopped, or 1 heaping TB. dried

2 TB. apple cider vinegar

1. In a 5½-quart slow cooker, add lentils, pearled barley, carrots, celery, yellow onion, garlic, basil, oregano, thyme, bay leaf, water, and chicken stock. Cover and cook on high for 6 to 8 hours.

2. 30 minutes before serving, stir in parsley and apple cider vinegar.

3. Turn off slow cooker, remove bay leaf, and serve piping hot.

PHABULOUS PHACT

Lentils are nearly a perfect food! Packed with one of the highest contents of both soluble and insoluble fiber, they're also a super source of molybdenum and folate; an excellent source of manganese; and a very good source of iron, protein, phosphorus, copper, thiamin, and potassium. They're a superior and inexpensive source of nutrition.

Cream of Carrot Soup

The warming flavors of ginger and black pepper complement the sweetness and comfort of carrots and potatoes in this creamy soup.

Yield:	Prep time:	Cook time:	Serving size:
7 cups	10 minutes	15 minutes	1 cup

Each serving has:			
28g carbohydrate	6g fat	4g fiber	7g protein

2 TB. olive oil

1 medium yellow onion, diced

4 large carrots, chopped

2 medium russet potatoes, peeled and chopped

2 tsp. fresh ginger, finely minced

1 cup water

3 cups almond or soy milk

1 tsp. sea salt

2 TB. fresh dill, finely chopped

¼ tsp. freshly ground black pepper

2 TB. fresh parsley, finely chopped

1 sheet sushi nori, cut into 2×⅛-in. strips

1. In a heavy-bottomed Dutch oven or stockpot over medium heat, heat olive oil. Add yellow onion, and sauté for 2 or 3 minutes.

2. Add carrots, russet potatoes, ginger, water, almond milk, and sea salt. Cover and simmer for 10 minutes or until vegetables are tender. Do not allow to boil (almond milk could curdle).

3. Using an immersion blender, purée soup until smooth.

4. Simmer for 5 more minutes, and serve either hot or chilled, garnished with parsley and nori strips.

BALANCE BONUS

This soup is especially delicious when served with a sprinkle of ground cinnamon or nutmeg. It makes the perfect accompaniment to a fall or winter holiday meal.

Curried Chickpea and Spinach Stew

The warm flavors and aromas of this healthfully balanced stew echo those of exotic India.

Yield:	Prep time:	Cook time:	Serving size:
4 cups	10 minutes	10 minutes	1 cup
Each serving has:			
24g carbohydrate	10g fat	8g fiber	10g protein

1 TB. olive oil

1 clove garlic, minced

¼ cup yellow onion, minced

1 (14.5-oz.) can diced tomatoes with green chiles, with juice

1 (15-oz.) can organic chickpeas, with juice, or 1½ cups cooked dried chickpeas

2 tsp. mild curry powder

⅓ cup unsweetened dried, flaked coconut

½ tsp. sea salt

6 cups fresh baby spinach leaves

2 cups cooked organic brown rice

2 TB. fresh parsley, minced

1. In a large saucepan over medium heat, heat olive oil. Add garlic and yellow onion, and sauté for 2 or 3 minutes or until soft, being careful not to brown garlic.

2. Add diced tomatoes with green chiles with juice, chickpeas, curry powder, coconut, and sea salt. Cover, bring to a boil, and cook over medium heat for 10 minutes.

3. Stir in baby spinach leaves, cover, reduce heat to low, and simmer for 2 or 3 more minutes or until spinach has turned bright green.

4. Serve hot over a bed of cooked brown rice, garnished with parsley.

PHABULOUS PHACT

Unlike commercially available curry powder, an authentic curry powder is made of up to 20 spices, herbs, and seeds. The most common components include cardamom, chiles, cinnamon, cloves, coriander, cumin, curry leaf, fennel seed, fenugreek, mace, mustard seed, nutmeg, poppy seed, saffron, sesame seed, tamarind, and turmeric.

Italian Fish Stew

The freshness of cucumber and sweetness of mace lighten this classic fish stew.

Yield:	Prep time:	Cook time:	Serving size:
6 cups	15 minutes	25 minutes	1½ cups
Each serving has:			
2.7g carbohydrate	7.1g fat	0g fiber	18.5g protein

2 TB. olive oil	1 tsp. sea salt
1 small white onion, thinly sliced	¼ tsp. coarsely ground black pepper
3 cloves garlic, smashed but not minced	⅛ tsp. mace
½ cup fresh parsley, chopped	½ cup water
½ medium cucumber, chopped	1 lb. fresh white-fleshed skinless fish fillets, cut into 4 thick portions
2 or 3 medium tomatoes, chopped	
2 bay leaves	

1. In a heavy-bottomed Dutch oven over medium heat, heat olive oil. Add white onion, garlic, parsley, cucumber, tomatoes, and bay leaves, and cook for 5 to 10 minutes or until vegetables have been well smothered.

2. Stir in sea salt, black pepper, mace, and water, and simmer, stirring occasionally, over medium heat for 20 minutes. If sauce becomes too thick, stir in a little more water.

3. Add fish fillets to sauce, and cook for about 5 more minutes or until fish is opaque and easily flakes with a fork.

4. Serve hot, garnished with additional parsley if desired.

PHABULOUS PHACT

Mace is the thin, delicately flavored covering on the shell of a nutmeg kernel. Both spices have been used in traditional medicines for their antidepressant, antifungal, aphrodisiac, carminative, and digestive properties.

Potato and Leek Soup

This velvety soup is a tasty alkalizing version of the French classic *vichyssoise*. You won't miss the lack of butter and heavy dairy cream.

Yield:	Prep time:	Cook time:	Serving size:
10 cups	15 minutes	1 hour	2 cups
Each serving has:			
26.6g carbohydrate	0.3g fat	3.9g fiber	2.9g protein

1 or 2 leeks, trimmed, sliced in half lengthwise, and tender green and white parts cut into ½-in. half-moons

3 or 4 medium russet potatoes, peeled and cubed

8 cups water

1 TB. sea salt

¼ tsp. coarsely ground black pepper

2 TB. fresh parsley, chopped

2 TB. fresh chives, chopped

1. Place leeks in a bowl of cool water, and swish around to thoroughly clean. Leeks will float, and any sand will sink to the bottom of the bowl.

2. In a heavy-bottomed Dutch oven over medium-high heat, combine russet potatoes, water, sea salt, and black pepper. Bring to a boil, reduce heat to medium-low, and simmer for about 15 minutes or until potatoes are tender.

3. Mash potatoes through a colander or food mill, return to water, and stir.

4. Remove leeks from water, and add to the Dutch oven. Add parsley, and stir to combine. Cook for about 40 more minutes or until leeks are tender and bright green.

5. Serve in soup bowls, hot or chilled, garnished with fresh chives.

DEFINITION

Vichyssoise is a classic puréed French soup made of leeks, potatoes, butter, cream, and chicken stock. It's usually served cold. When it's served warm, it's known as *potage parmentier.* If it's made without dairy, it's called *potage bonne femme.*

Veggies, Grains, and Legumes

In This Chapter

- pH-balancing vegetable dishes
- Great grain recipes
- Protein-rich legume dishes

Vegetables form the foundation of the pH balance diet. Simply prepared raw or freshly juiced vegetables should form a large portion of your pH balance diet, but the cooked veggie dishes in this chapter will add variety and interest to your menus. With their low calorie content, you can feel free to fill up on them, too.

Grains and legumes also are important in the pH balance diet. Examine the tables in Appendix C, and you might notice that most grains and legumes fall in the mildly to moderately acid-forming category. But that doesn't tell the whole story. Grains and legumes are rich sources of vitamins and minerals and an important source of protein. While on the pH balance diet, you usually limit or omit red meats and fish, so grains and legumes are an excellent way to get the protein you need.

Stand-Out Stuffed Tomatoes

A spicy note of roasted eggplant pairs with the sweetness of zucchini and fresh spinach in this very-vegetable stuffed-tomato dish.

Yield:	Prep time:	Cook time:	Serving size:
4 stuffed tomato halves	10 minutes	30 minutes	1 stuffed tomato half

Each serving has:			
4.8g carbohydrate	3.8g fat	1.3g fiber	1.1g protein

2 very large fresh tomatoes, halved along their equator	1/2 medium yellow onion, diced medium
1/2 small eggplant, peeled and diced medium	1 clove garlic, minced
	1/4 tsp. sea salt
1/2 small zucchini, diced	1/8 tsp. coarsely ground black pepper
1 cup handful fresh baby spinach, roughly chopped	
	1 TB. olive oil

1. Preheat the oven to 350°F.

2. Scoop out seeds and soft inner pulp from tomatoes and add to a medium bowl. Set aside tomato shells.

3. Add eggplant, zucchini, spinach, yellow onion, garlic, sea salt, black pepper, and olive oil to the bowl, and mix well.

4. Stuff each tomato shell with as much vegetable mixture as will fit, mounding it up in the center if necessary, and place stuffed shells in a shallow baking dish. Add about 1/4 inch water in the bottom of the pan.

5. Cover the dish tightly with aluminum foil, and roast for 30 minutes.

6. Carefully remove foil—steam will escape. Remove tomatoes from the pan using a slotted spoon or spatula, and serve.

BALANCE BONUS

For a very alkalinizing lunch or light meal, divide this recipe into two servings—2 stuffed shells each—and serve with a fresh garden salad.

Alkalizing Steam-Fried Veggies

Warm, steam-fried vegetables and sprouts offer a burst of fresh garden flavor to any meal.

Yield:	Prep time:	Cook time:	Serving size:
4 cups	10 minutes	10 minutes	1 cup

Each serving has:			
40.4g carbohydrate	0.8g fat	6.1g fiber	16.9g protein

$\frac{1}{4}$ cup water

1 clove garlic, minced

$\frac{1}{2}$ large head broccoli, broken into small florets

$\frac{1}{2}$ large head cauliflower, cut or broken into small florets

1 medium red bell pepper, ribs and seeds removed, and sliced into $\frac{1}{4}$-in. strips

Handful raw mung bean sprouts, rinsed

Handful raw alfalfa sprouts, rinsed

1 cup cooked wild rice or brown basmati rice

3 medium green onions, white and green parts, sliced

Bragg Liquid Aminos or naturally fermented soy sauce

1. In a medium skillet over medium heat, bring water to a boil. Add garlic, and steam-fry for 3 minutes or until softened.

2. Add broccoli, cauliflower, red bell pepper, mung bean sprouts, and alfalfa sprouts, and cook, stirring, for about 3 to 5 more minutes or until vegetables have been heated through.

3. Add cooked rice and green onions, and cook, stirring, until rice has been thoroughly warmed through.

4. Spoon vegetable–rice mixture onto a serving platter, spritz vegetables with 2 or 3 sprays of Bragg Liquid Aminos, lightly toss, and serve.

Bragg Liquid Aminos is a salty-flavored dietary supplement often used for seasoning foods. The product is a certified non-GMO (genetically modified organism), gluten-free liquid protein concentrate derived from soybeans that contains the essential and conditionally essential amino acids in naturally occurring amounts, without the use of chemicals, artificial coloring, alcohol, or preservatives.

Red Radish Delight

Raw radishes have a sharp, spicy flavor, but when cooked, they become delightfully reminiscent of sweet, creamed turnips.

Yield:	Prep time:	Cook time:	Serving size:
4 cups	5 minutes	5 minutes	1 cup

Each serving has:			
9g carbohydrate	0g fat	3g fiber	1g protein

2 cups whole red radishes with tops

2 cups water

2 umeboshi plums, pitted

1 tsp. ume plum vinegar

3 TB. kuzu root starch, dissolved in 4 TB. cold water

1. Bring a small saucepan half-full of water to a boil over medium-high heat.

2. Wash and trim radishes and their greens, reserving greens.

3. In a medium saucepan over medium-high heat, combine radishes, 2 cups water, umeboshi plums, and ume plum vinegar. Cover, bring to a boil, reduce heat to medium-low, and simmer for 5 minutes.

4. Meanwhile, quickly blanch radish greens in the small saucepan of boiling water for 2 minutes. Set aside greens until they're cool enough to handle.

5. Using your hands, squeeze water from blanched greens and roughly chop. Place in a serving dish.

6. Remove umeboshi plums from the saucepan, and discard. Using a slotted spoon, remove radishes, and place them in the serving dish. Toss lightly with greens.

7. Whisk kuzu mixture into cooking liquid, and cook, whisking constantly, for 3 more minutes or until sauce becomes thick and translucent.

8. Spoon sauce over radishes and greens, and serve warm.

BALANCE BONUS

If you can't find radishes with their greens intact, substitute a small bunch of fresh turnip greens.

Roasted Vegetable Medley

This versatile vegetable dish is a healthy addition to any meal, and the leftovers make a wonderfully flavorful breakfast the next morning.

Yield:	Prep time:	Cook time:	Serving size:
8 cups	15 minutes	45 minutes	1 cup

Each serving has:			
48g carbohydrate	8g fat	9g fiber	4g protein

6 cloves garlic, separated	2 large yellow onions, quartered
5 medium parsnips, trimmed and cut into 1-in. chunks	1 medium butternut squash, peeled, seeded, and cubed
4 medium white or red potatoes, skin on, scrubbed and cubed	4 TB. olive oil
2 medium sweet potatoes, skin on, scrubbed and cubed	1 tsp. sea salt

1. Preheat the oven to 400°F. Line a large baking sheet with aluminum foil, and lightly grease the foil.

2. In a large bowl, combine garlic, parsnips, potatoes, sweet potatoes, yellow onions, and butternut squash. Add olive oil, and toss to coat.

3. Spread vegetables in an even layer on the prepared baking sheet, and sprinkle with sea salt. Roast for 35 to 45 minutes or until vegetables are tender and slightly browned.

4. Serve immediately.

BALANCE BONUS

Including plenty of root vegetables, winter squash, and leafy green vegetables in your diet goes a long way toward balancing the pH of your meals. The vegetables in this recipe have an abundance of alkalizing minerals such as potassium, calcium, magnesium, and manganese.

Onion Wakame Casserole

Onions and carrots bring a great deal of sweetness to this healthful vegetarian casserole.

Yield:	Prep time:	Cook time:	Serving size:
4 cups	15 minutes	40 minutes	1 cup

Each serving has:			
14g carbohydrate	6g fat	4g fiber	4g protein

2 tsp. shoyu soy sauce, or to taste

5 TB. organic tahini

2 cups water

3 or 4 medium yellow onions, thinly sliced (about 4 cups)

2 pieces wakame, soaked in cold water to cover for 5 minutes, drained, and roughly chopped

1 large carrot, julienned (1 cup)

1. Preheat the oven to 350°F.

2. In a large bowl, combine shoyu soy sauce, tahini, and water. Add onions, wakame, and carrot, and toss thoroughly.

3. Place mixture in a small casserole dish, cover, and bake for 40 to 45 minutes or until onions are tender.

4. Serve immediately.

PHABULOUS PHACT

Onions, garlic, leeks, and chives are members of the allium family and are rich in the sulfur-containing compounds responsible for their distinctive flavors, aromas, and many of their health-promoting attributes. These plants promote cardiovascular health, provide support to bone and connective tissues, are anti-inflammatory, and have been found to aid in cancer prevention.

Old-Fashioned Scalloped Potatoes

For flavor, warmth, and comfort, scalloped potatoes can't be beat—and they do a phenomenal job of balancing pH in meals.

Yield:	Prep time:	Cook time:	Serving size:
2 quarts	10 minutes	1 hour	1⅓ cups
Each serving has:			
35g carbohydrate	7g fat	5g fiber	4g protein

3 TB. ghee

3 TB. *spelt* flour

1 tsp. sea salt

¼ tsp. freshly ground black pepper

2½ cups unsweetened almond milk

6 medium russet potatoes, peeled and thinly sliced

1 medium yellow onion, thinly sliced

1. Preheat the oven to 350°F. Lightly grease a 3-quart casserole dish, and set aside.

2. In a medium saucepan over medium heat, make a light roux by heating ghee while whisking in spelt flour, sea salt, and black pepper. Continue to cook, continuously stirring, for about 5 minutes or until roux is completely smooth and bubbly but not browned.

3. Whisk in almond milk, ½ cup at a time, ensuring each addition is thoroughly combined before adding more. Continue stirring, bring to a boil, and boil for 1 minute. Remove from heat.

4. Add russet potatoes and yellow onion to the casserole dish in three layers: arrange ⅓ of potatoes in the bottom of the dish, topped by ⅓ of onions and ⅓ of sauce. Repeat these layers twice.

5. Cover casserole, and bake for about 45 minutes or until potatoes are tender.

6. Uncover and bake for 10 to 15 more minutes or until edges are nicely brown and crispy.

7. Let rest for 10 minutes to thicken before serving.

> **PHABULOUS PHACT**
>
> Potatoes originated in Peru more than 4 millennia ago, and approximately 4,000 varieties are still grown there. Potatoes are an excellent source of pH-balancing potassium and vitamin C.

Vegetable Sushi Rolls

This vegetable sushi roll, made with creamy avocado, crunchy cucumber, and sweet carrots, has a few secret ingredients: snappy sprouts, lively green onion, and the freshness of dill.

Yield:	Prep time:	Serving size:	
4 sushi rolls	15 minutes, plus 1 hour chill time	1 sushi roll, sliced	
Each serving has:			
85g carbohydrate	13g fat	11g fiber	11g protein

4 sushi nori sheets

2 medium Hass avocados, mashed (2 cups)

2 cups cooked brown rice

1 medium cucumber, julienned

2 medium carrots, shredded (1 cup)

1 cup sprouted alfalfa, clover, or broccoli seeds, or a combination

1 cup shredded cabbage

1 medium green onion, green parts only, thinly sliced

3 sprigs fresh dill, chopped

1. Place nori sheets on a flat surface, shiny side down. Leaving a 1-inch border, spread avocado evenly on nori sheets. In a horizontal line across center of each sheet, place a row of brown rice, cucumber, carrots, alfalfa sprouts, cabbage, green onion, and dill.

2. Beginning at the edge closest to you, firmly roll nori sheet into a log. Wrap rolls in plastic wrap, and refrigerate for 1 hour to increase firmness.

3. Unwrap rolls from plastic and, using a sharp knife, slice into 1-inch-thick portions. Arrange on plates, flat side down, and serve.

BALANCE BONUS

The popular California roll typically has avocado, kani kama (imitation crab), and cucumber, and it's often served uramaki style (with rice on the outside and nori on the inside). Western takes on sushi such as this one are rarely found in Japan, but they're just as healthy and flavorfully tailored to the Western palate. Have fun experimenting with sushi using some of your own favorite flavor combinations, such as radish, herbed mayonnaise, tuna, chiles, salmon, lettuce, and even scrambled egg.

Zucchini and Quinoa with Chickpea Sauce

Garden-fresh zucchini combines with earthy chickpeas and hearty quinoa for an excellent side dish or quick and easy vegetarian meal.

Yield:	Prep time:	Cook time:	Serving size:
8 cups	5 minutes	20 minutes	2 cups

Each serving has:			
155g carbohydrate	28g fat	40g fiber	47g protein

1 cup quinoa	4 TB. extra-virgin olive oil
2 cups plus 2 TB. water	$\frac{1}{2}$ tsp. chili powder
2 (15-oz.) cans organic chickpeas, rinsed and drained	$\frac{1}{2}$ tsp. ground cumin
1 large tomato, roughly chopped	$\frac{1}{4}$ lb. silken tofu (about $\frac{1}{4}$ block)
1 clove garlic, minced	4 medium zucchini, sliced on the bias
1 TB. freshly squeezed lemon juice	1 handful fresh cilantro, torn
	2 TB. sesame seeds

1. In a medium saucepan over medium-high heat, bring quinoa and 2 cups water to a boil. Reduce heat to low, cover, and simmer for 10 minutes or until all water has been absorbed. Set aside.

2. In a blender, process chickpeas, tomato, garlic, lemon juice, 2 tablespoons extra-virgin olive oil, chili powder, cumin, and tofu until smooth and creamy.

3. In a medium skillet over medium-high heat, heat remaining 2 tablespoons water. Add zucchini, and steam-fry for about 3 to 5 minutes or until tender-crisp.

4. Add chickpea mixture, stir, and cook for 2 or 3 more minutes or until heated through.

5. Stir in 1 tablespoon extra-virgin olive oil, and remove from heat.

6. Divide quinoa between 2 plates, top with zucchini sauce, garnish with cilantro and sesame seeds, drizzle with remaining 1 tablespoon extra-virgin olive oil, and serve.

PHABULOUS PHACT

Recipes calling for tofu usually indicate what type to use—silken, firm, extra firm, for example. If not, it's safest to stick with firm. Firmer tofu is recommended for stir-fries and grilling, while soft tofu works well in soups, and silken tofu is great for blended dishes like sauces, puddings, and purées.

Yummy Millet Mash

The nutty taste and unique texture of millet combines with mildly flavorful cauliflower to make an interesting alternative to standard starchy sides like potatoes and rice.

Yield:	Prep time:	Cook time:	Serving size:
4 cups	5 minutes	30 minutes	1 cup
Each serving has:			
40g carbohydrate	2g fat	6g fiber	7g protein

1 cup millet
2½ cups water
Pinch sea salt

1 small head cauliflower, thinly sliced
¼ cup fresh parsley, chopped

1. Rinse millet well, and drain.

2. In a medium saucepan over medium-high heat, bring millet, water, and salt to a boil. Add cauliflower, and return to a boil. Reduce heat to low, and simmer for 20 minutes or until water has been absorbed and millet is tender. Remove from heat.

3. Using a potato masher, mash millet and cauliflower.

4. Fold in parsley, and serve.

> **BALANCE BONUS**
>
> Always rinse grains and legumes before cooking to remove any natural debris that might remain after processing and packaging. Be sure to rinse quinoa very well to remove the bitter saponin coating. Run water over quinoa until no soaplike suds remain when you swish the seed around with your hands. When the rinse water runs clear, the saponins are gone.

Tarka Dhal (Indian Spiced Lentils)

Exotic flavors and aromas of India, defined by garlic, chiles, turmeric, and cumin, highlight this traditional Indian dish.

Yield:	Prep time:	Cook time:	Serving size:
4 cups	5 minutes	40 minutes	1 cup

Each serving has:			
28g carbohydrate	6g fat	12g fiber	10g protein

1 TB. ghee or unsalted butter	3¼ cups water
1 medium yellow onion, chopped	¾ cup split red lentils
2 cloves garlic, minced	1 tsp. ground turmeric
2 dried red chiles, coarsely chopped	1 tsp. ground cumin
	1 tsp. sea salt

1. In a medium skillet over medium heat, melt ghee. Add yellow onion, garlic, and red chilies, and sauté for 5 minutes or until onion has turned golden brown. Set aside.

2. In a medium saucepan over medium-high heat, bring water, split red lentils, turmeric, cumin, and sea salt to a boil. Reduce heat to medium, and cook, stirring, for 10 minutes.

3. Cover and simmer lentils for 30 more minutes.

4. Remove the saucepan from heat, and allow to cool slightly.

5. Using an immersion blender, make a slight purée of cooked lentils, or process about half of lentils in a blender and return to the saucepan.

6. Stir in half of onion mixture.

7. Spoon lentils into a serving dish, garnish with remaining onion mixture, and serve.

PHABULOUS PHACT

Lentils have been cultivated since about 6000 B.C.E. in the Middle East, where they were traditionally eaten with barley or wheat. From there, their use spread widely throughout Africa and Asia. By the first century, they had been introduced into India's cuisine, where a spiced lentil dish, *dhal,* is always included as part of a meal, even today.

Delectable Desserts

In This Chapter

- pH-balancing desserts
- Fresh and fruity desserts
- Fun, frozen sweet tooth tamers
- Crave-worthy chocolate desserts

The sugar, refined flours, and artificial ingredients found in many desserts can be highly acidifying, and you might think sweets are an automatic no-no on the pH balance diet. Not so fast. In the same way you need to plan to have healthy snacks available, you also should have a plan for those special occasions when nothing but dessert will do. Otherwise, you'll find yourself caught off guard when birthdays, anniversaries, and other dessert-worthy occasions come around.

Because the desserts in this chapter make good use of alkalizing ingredients, they have a minimal impact on pH. They're not very alkalizing, but they're not terribly acidifying, either. If reserved for a weekly treat, or for times when true celebration is in order, these delectable dessert recipes will help keep your diet on track while you indulge just a little bit. Remember, if you eat alkalizing foods 80 to 90 percent of the time, you can afford to treat yourself now and then!

Lemon Chiffon Cake

Lovely lemon juice, tofu, and chickpea flour work magic to make this cake an occasional special treat.

Yield:	Prep time:	Cook time:	Serving size:
1 (8×4-inch) cake	10 minutes	30 minutes	1 (½-inch) slice

Each serving has:			
24.1g carbohydrate	0.5g fat	5.2g fiber	8.5g protein

1 cup chickpea flour	Zest of 2 medium lemons
2 tsp. baking powder	Juice of 2 medium lemons
1 (12-oz.) pkg. firm tofu	2 TB. water
3 TB. agave syrup	

1. Preheat the oven to 350°F. Grease an 8×4-inch loaf pan, or line it with a sheet of parchment paper.

2. In a small bowl, combine chickpea flour and baking powder. Set aside.

3. In a medium bowl, and using an electric mixer on medium speed, combine tofu, agave syrup, lemon zest, and lemon juice for about 5 minutes or until batter is very creamy and light.

4. Continue mixing for 5 more minutes while incorporating flour mixture to wet mixture ¼ cup at a time.

5. Pour batter into the prepared pan, and bake for 25 to 30 minutes. Cake will be slightly springy but firm when done.

6. Remove cake from the oven, and allow to cool completely in the pan on a wire rack for about 30 minutes.

7. Remove cake from the pan by turning it out or lifting it with the parchment paper. Slice in ½-inch slices, and serve.

BALANCE BONUS

This is a perfect cake to make ahead and freeze. Wrapped securely in plastic wrap, it will stay fresh and be ready to serve the next time unexpected guests arrive. Make some lemony herbal iced tea to serve with it, and you can treat your guests to a balanced dessert without batting an eye!

Cranberry Crumble

The tart flavor of cranberries provides a unique freshness to this not-too-sweet dessert.

Yield:	Prep time:	Cook time:	Serving size:
1 (8- or 9-inch) crumble	5 minutes	30 minutes	¼ of crumble

Each serving has:			
19.8g carbohydrate	0g fat	2.3g fiber	1.7g protein

1 cup fresh or frozen cranberries	½ cup old-fashioned rolled oats
2 TB. agave syrup	1 TB. millet flour
1 cup water	

1. Preheat the oven to 350°F.

2. In a small saucepan over medium heat, cook cranberries, 1 tablespoon agave syrup, and water until cranberries burst. Pour mixture into a (8- or 9-inch) pie pan, and set aside.

3. In a medium bowl, combine old-fashioned rolled oats and millet flour. Add remaining 1 tablespoon agave syrup, and mix well.

4. Evenly sprinkle crumbly oat and flour mixture over top of cranberries, and bake for about 15 minutes or until top is crisp and slightly browned.

5. Allow to rest for 5 minutes before serving.

PHABULOUS PHACT

Although cranberries are considered an acid-forming food, they have a special place in any healthy diet. Cranberries promote urinary tract health, are high in vitamin C, and are valuable for reducing pain and inflammation. If you're going to eat cranberries on the pH balance diet, remember to reserve them for special occasions.

Baked Fruit Southern Comfort

Baked apples or pears are naturally sweet and oh-so-satisfying!

Yield:	Prep time:	Cook time:	Serving size:
4 baked apples or pears	1 minute	20 minutes	1 apple or pear
Each serving has:			
31g carbohydrate	0g fat	5g fiber	0.5g protein

4 medium to large apples or
　　pears, cored

1. Preheat the oven to 400°F.

2. Place apples in an ovenproof baking dish, and bake for 15 to 20 minutes or until apples have softened.

3. Serve immediately on dessert plates drizzled with pan juices.

> **PHABULOUS PHACT**
>
> Several cancer studies have shown that consuming apples daily provides cancer-preventive benefits. So there may be some truth to the adage "An apple a day keeps the doctor away!"

Strawberry Sorbet

Bright and tangy-sweet, there's nothing like an icy fruit sorbet on a hot summer day.

Yield:	Prep time:	Serving size:	
1 quart	40 minutes	1 cup	
Each serving has:			
29.5g carbohydrate	1.3g fat	2.3g fiber	1g protein

1 lb. fresh strawberries, hulled
2 TB. agave syrup

2 cups rice milk
Mint leaves

1. In a blender or a food processor fitted with a chopping blade, purée strawberries.

2. Add agave syrup and rice milk, and process for about 1 more minute.

3. Pour sorbet base into an ice cream maker, and churn for 30 minutes.

4. Scoop sorbet onto individual dessert plates, garnish with mint leaves, and serve immediately.

BALANCE BONUS

If you don't own an ice cream maker, you can still make your own sorbet. Place the sorbet base in a shallow freezer container, and whisk the contents every half hour until the sorbet has frozen.

Fresh Fruit Granita

Let this mango ice treat transport your taste buds straight to a sunny tropical paradise.

Yield:	Prep time:	Serving size:	
3 cups	40 minutes	¾ cup	
Each serving has:			
19.4g carbohydrate	0.3g fat	2.3g fiber	0.7g protein

2 medium ripe mangoes, peeled and pitted

Juice of 1 medium lime

½ cup cold water

Red grapes or currants

1. In a blender or a food processor fitted with a chopping blade, process mango until smooth.

2. Add lime juice and water, and process for a few more seconds until thoroughly incorporated.

3. Pour mixture into an ice cream maker, and churn for 30 minutes.

4. Serve immediately in pretty stemmed glasses, garnished with red grapes or currants.

BALANCE BONUS

This granita will keep well frozen for up to a month. Make up a batch to have on hand the next time you find mangoes.

Watermelon Berry Floats

This cool and refreshing fruity float is the perfect dessert for hot summer afternoons.

Yield:	Prep time:	Serving size:	
2 floats (2 cups fruit plus 2 scoops sorbet)	5 minutes	1 float (1 cup fruit plus 1 scoop sorbet)	
Each serving has:			
39g carbohydrate	.4g fat	2g fiber	1g protein

1 cup (½-in.) watermelon cubes

1 cup strawberries, roughly chopped

1 tsp. balsamic vinegar

⅛ tsp. cayenne

2 scoops citrus sorbet (about ½ cup)

Sparkling mineral water or club soda, chilled

2 sprigs fresh mint

1. In a medium bowl, toss together watermelon cubes, strawberries, balsamic vinegar, and cayenne.

2. Place ¼ of fruit mixture in the bottom of each of 2 tall glasses. Top each with 1 scoop citrus sorbet.

3. Evenly divide remaining fruit mixture between the glasses, drizzling any juice from the bowl over top.

4. Fill each glass with sparkling mineral water, garnish with mint and additional fruit, if desired, and serve immediately.

PHABULOUS PHACT

Watermelon is a diuretic fruit made up of 92 percent water. It's useful for balancing pH, helping flush the kidneys, fighting water retention, and providing a naturally sweet treat suitable even for diabetics and others who are sugar sensitive.

Chocolate Tofu Mousse

This fabulous mousse made with soy milk and silken tofu tastes every bit as decadent as the original French version!

Yield:	Prep time:	Cook time:	Serving size:
3¾ cups	10 minutes, plus 1 hour chill time	5 minutes	¾ cup

Each serving has:			
30g carbohydrate	18.6g fat	5g fiber	6g protein

8 oz. bittersweet chocolate, chopped	10 oz. silken tofu, drained
1 cup soy milk	½ cup mixed fresh berries of choice
½ vanilla bean, scraped	

1. Place chopped bittersweet chocolate in a bowl, and set aside.

2. In a medium saucepan over medium-high heat, combine soy milk and vanilla bean, and bring to a boil.

3. Pour soy milk mixture over bittersweet chocolate, and allow to stand for 1 minute. Remove and discard vanilla bean pod, and whisk mixture until smooth.

4. In a blender, process silken tofu for about 10 or 15 seconds or until creamy. Add chocolate mixture, and blend for about 30 more seconds or until smooth.

5. Spoon mousse into bowls and refrigerate for about 1 hour or until firm.

6. Evenly divide mixed berries among bowls as a topping, and serve chilled.

PHABULOUS PHACT

Mousse is a French word that means "foam," so *Mousse au Chocolat* means "chocolate foam." In 1894, when mousses first became all the rage in culinary circles, they were made of savory ingredients such as seafood and vegetables. Everything changed, however, when, in the 1900s, French painter Henri de Toulouse-Lautrec discovered that, by using chocolate, he could create the delightfully light and creamy dessert we know today.

Crazy-for-Chocolate Dessert Sauce

The dark chocolate and mocha flavors of this dessert sauce turn even a plain bowl of fresh berries into a celebratory repast.

Yield:	Prep time:	Cook time:	Serving size:
1¾ cups	5 minutes	5 minutes	¼ cup

Each serving has:			
25g carbohydrate	4.2g fat	2g fiber	1g protein

2½ oz. bittersweet chocolate, chopped small

⅓ cup unsweetened cocoa powder

¼ cup dark brown sugar, firmly packed

1 tsp. organic instant coffee granules, or grain beverage substitute

1 cup water

¼ cup agave syrup

2½ tsp. vanilla extract

1. In a blender or a food processor fitted with a chopping blade, process bittersweet chocolate, cocoa powder, dark brown sugar, and instant coffee granules for about 1 minute or until finely ground. Set aside, but do not remove contents from blender.

2. In a small saucepan over medium-high heat, heat water. Stir in agave syrup, and bring to a slow boil.

3. With the blender running, pour in agave syrup mixture and vanilla extract. Process until sauce is smooth, scraping down the sides, if necessary.

4. Serve warm immediately, or transfer to an airtight container and refrigerate for about 2 hours or until chilled. Stir before serving.

BALANCE BONUS

Although this is a sweet dessert sauce, the sweeteners are put to good use. Sweetening this rich sauce with brown sugar, agave syrup, and vanilla extract reduces the number of "empty" calories, providing nutrition along with important antioxidants and 17 milligrams alkalizing calcium!

Glossary

acid A chemical substance possessing a value of less than 7 on the pH scale. Acids are proton donors that have the ability to neutralize alkaline solutions (bases).

acidogenic Acid producing; an acidogenic diet is one made of foods that increase the body's level of acidity.

acidosis A state indicated by excessive acid accumulation in the body's tissues, especially the blood.

adenosine triphosphate (ATP) A vital cellular fuel synthesized within cells from glucose and oxygen. ATP is integral for healthy cell metabolism and replication.

adipose tissue A type of body tissue that contains stored cellular fat, serves as a source of energy, cushions and insulates vital organs, and is active in the formation of hormones.

alkali A chemical substance with a value greater than 7 on the pH scale. Alkaline substances, or bases, are proton acceptors and have the ability to neutralize acidic solutions.

alkalosis A state indicated by excessive accumulation of alkalinity in the body's tissues, especially the blood.

allspice A spice named for its flavor echoes of several spices (cinnamon, cloves, nutmeg) used in many desserts and in rich marinades and stews.

amaranth An ancient high-protein (12 to 17 percent) grain that can be used whole, ground into flour for use in baked goods, popped like popcorn, or flaked like oatmeal. Amaranth has been shown to reduce cholesterol.

amino acids   The nitrogen-containing building blocks from which proteins are made.

anaerobic respiration   A form of cellular respiration that occurs when oxygen is absent or scarce.

antioxidant   A substance that reduces damaging oxidation caused by free radicals. Antioxidants reduce the risk of cancer and the development of age-related diseases. Well-known antioxidants include vitamins C and E.

arborio rice   A plump Italian rice used for, among other purposes, risotto.

artichoke heart   The center part of the artichoke flower, often found canned in grocery stores.

arugula   A spicy-peppery green with leaves that resemble a dandelion and have a distinctive and very sharp flavor.

Ayurvedic medicine   Sometimes called Ayurveda, this is one of the world's oldest medical systems, developed and evolved over thousands of years in India. Ayurveda employs the use of herbs and specially tailored diets and techniques designed to balance the body, mind, and spirit.

baba ghanoush   A traditional Middle Eastern eggplant dish typically served with warm pita bread and an assortment of crudités.

bake   To cook in a dry oven.

baking powder   A dry ingredient used to increase volume and lighten or leaven baked goods.

balsamic vinegar   Vinegar produced primarily in Italy from a specific type of grape and aged in wood barrels. It's heavier, darker, and sweeter than most vinegars.

basil   A flavorful, almost sweet, resinous herb delicious with tomatoes and used in all kinds of Italian- and Mediterranean-style dishes.

baste   To keep foods moist during cooking by spooning, brushing, or drizzling with a liquid.

Belgian endive   *See* endive.

bilayer   The self-aligning structure that forms the interior and exterior boundary of a cell. It's made of pairs of phospholipids that have a hydrophobic tail and hydrophilic head.

bioflavonoid   Once known as vitamin P, this is the class of plant metabolites found in the natural pigments in fruits and vegetables. Three of the flavonoid classes are ketone-containing compounds that show much promise in preventing and mitigating neurodegenerative disease states such as the various dementias, MS, ALS, and Parkinson's disease.

blanch   To place a food in boiling water for about 1 minute or less to partially cook the exterior and then submerge in or rinse with cool water to halt the cooking.

body mass index (BMI)   A relative measure of ideal weight determined by using one of the following formulas:

$$\text{English: BMI} = [\text{weight in pounds} / (\text{height in inches})]^2 \times 703$$

$$\text{Metric: BMI} = \text{weight in kilograms} / (\text{height in meters})^2$$

bok choy   A member of the cabbage family with thick stems, crisp texture, and fresh flavor. It's perfect for stir-frying.

bonito flakes   Preserved skipjack tuna that's been steamed, dried, and shaved into flakes for use as a salty-flavored seasoning.

bouillon   Dried essence of stock from chicken, beef, vegetables, or other ingredients. It's a popular starting ingredient for soups because it adds flavor (and often a lot of salt).

Bragg Liquid Aminos   A salty-flavored dietary supplement often used for seasoning foods. It's a certified non-GMO, gluten-free liquid protein concentrate derived from soybeans that contains the essential and conditionally essential amino acids in naturally occurring amounts, without chemicals, artificial coloring, alcohol, or preservatives.

braise   To cook with the introduction of some liquid, usually over an extended period of time.

broth   *See* stock.

brown   To cook in a skillet, turning, until the food's surface is seared and brown in color, to lock in the juices.

brown rice   A whole-grain rice, including the germ, with a characteristic pale brown or tan color. It's more nutritious and flavorful than white rice.

bruschetta (or crostini)   Slices of toasted or grilled bread with garlic and olive oil, often with other toppings.

buko juice   The clear liquid (coconut water) inside young coconuts.

bulgur   A wheat kernel that's been steamed, dried, and crushed and is sold in fine and coarse textures.

caper   The flavorful buds of a Mediterranean plant, ranging in size from *nonpareil* (about the size of a small pea) to larger, grape-size caper berries produced in Spain.

caramelize   To cook sugar over low heat until it develops a sweet caramel flavor, or to cook vegetables or meat in butter or oil over low heat until they soften, sweeten, and develop a caramel color.

caraway   A distinctive spicy seed used for bread, pork, cheese, and cabbage dishes. It's known to reduce stomach upset, which is why it's often paired with foods like sauerkraut.

cardamom   An intense, sweet-smelling spice used in baking and coffee, common in Indian cooking.

carob   A tropical tree that produces long pods from which the dried, baked, and powdered flesh—carob powder—is used in baking. The flavor is sweet and reminiscent of chocolate.

catabolic state   A state in which the body begins to break down its own tissues.

cayenne   A fiery spice made from hot chile peppers, especially the cayenne chile, a slender, red, and very hot pepper.

chevre   A creamy-salty soft goat cheese. Chevres vary in style from mild and creamy to aged, firm, and flavorful.

chickpea (or garbanzo bean) A roundish yellow-gold bean used as the base ingredient in hummus. Chickpeas are high in fiber and low in fat.

chile (or **chili**) Any one of many different "hot" peppers, ranging in intensity from the relatively mild ancho pepper to the blisteringly hot habanero.

chili powder A warm, rich seasoning blend that includes chile pepper, cumin, garlic, and oregano.

Chinese five-spice powder A pungent mixture of equal parts cinnamon, cloves, fennel seed, anise, and Szechuan peppercorns.

chipotle pepper A ripe, smoked jalapeño. Chipotles are an important spice in Mexican cuisine and give foods a medium to high heat and a complex, smoky flavor.

chive A member of the onion family, chives grow in bunches of long leaves that resemble tall grass or the green tops of onions and offer a light onion flavor.

chutney A thick condiment often served with Indian curries made with fruits and/or vegetables with vinegar, sugar, and spices.

cider vinegar A vinegar produced from apple cider, popular in North America.

cilantro A member of the parsley family used in Mexican dishes (especially salsa) and some Asian dishes. Use in moderation because the flavor can overwhelm. The seed of the cilantro plant is the spice coriander.

cinnamon A rich, aromatic spice commonly used in baking or desserts.

clove A sweet, strong, almost wintergreen-flavor spice used in baking.

coriander A rich, warm, spicy seed used in all types of recipes, from African to South American, from entrées to desserts.

couscous Granular semolina (durum wheat) that's cooked and used in many Mediterranean and North African dishes.

crimini mushroom   A relative of the white button mushroom that's brown in color and has a richer flavor. The larger, fully grown version is the portobello. *See also* portobello mushroom.

cumin   A fiery, smoky-tasting spice popular in Middle Eastern and Indian dishes. Cumin is a seed; ground cumin seed is the most common form used in cooking.

curry   Rich, spicy, Indian-style sauces and the dishes prepared with them. A curry uses curry powder as its base seasoning.

curry powder   A ground blend of rich and flavorful spices used as a basis for curry and many other Indian-influenced dishes. Common ingredients include hot pepper, nutmeg, cumin, cinnamon, pepper, and turmeric. Some curry can also be found in paste form.

custard   A cooked mixture of eggs and milk popular as a base for desserts.

daikon   Japanese for "large root," this is a large (up to 14 inches in length and 4 inches in diameter), mildly flavored white radish commonly used in Asian cuisines. It's commonly called mooli in Europe and continental Asia.

dash   A few drops, usually of a liquid, released by a quick shake.

deglaze   To scrape up bits of meat and seasoning left in a pan or skillet after cooking. Usually this is done by adding a liquid such as wine or broth and creating a flavorful stock that can be used to create sauces.

demineralization   The loss of vital minerals from the body's tissues, such as in osteoporosis. In states of chronic acidity, calcium, potassium, magnesium, and other alkalizing minerals may be pulled from the bones and other tissues and used as a buffer against acidity.

Dijon mustard   A hearty, spicy mustard made in the style of the Dijon region of France.

dill   An herb perfect for eggs, salmon, cheese dishes, and, of course, vegetables (pickles!).

double boiler   A set of two pots designed to nest together, one inside the other, and provide consistent, moist heat for foods that need delicate treatment. The bottom pot holds water (not quite touching the bottom of the top pot); the top pot holds the food you want to heat.

dredge   To coat a piece of food on all sides with a dry substance such as flour or cornmeal.

edamame   Fresh, plump, pale green soybeans, similar in appearance to lima beans, often served steamed and either shelled or still in their protective pods.

emulsion   A combination of liquid ingredients that don't normally mix well (such as a fat or oil with water) that are beaten together to create a thick liquid. Creating emulsions must be done carefully and rapidly to ensure that the particles of one ingredient are suspended in the other.

endive   A green that resembles a small, elongated, tightly packed head of romaine lettuce. The thick, crunchy leaves can be broken off and used with dips and spreads.

extra-virgin olive oil   *See* olive oil.

extract   A concentrated flavoring derived from foods or plants through evaporation or distillation that imparts a powerful flavor without altering the volume or texture of a dish.

falafel   A Middle Eastern food made of seasoned, ground chickpeas formed into balls, cooked, and often used as a filling in pitas.

fennel   In seed form, a fragrant, licorice-tasting herb. The bulbs have a mild flavor and a celery-like crunch and are used as a vegetable in salads or cooked recipes.

fold   To combine a dense and light mixture with a circular action from the middle of the bowl.

free radical   An unstable molecule that damages other molecules, which results in the formation of more free radicals. Free radicals are capable of damaging the body's tissues and setting the stage for various diseases.

frittata   A skillet-cooked mixture of eggs and other ingredients that's not stirred but is cooked slowly and then either flipped or finished under the broiler.

fry   *See* sauté.

Galia melon   The first hybrid melon created from intensely fragrant Middle Eastern melons. It looks like a cantaloupe on the outside and a honeydew on the inside. Its flesh is sweet tasting, smooth, and light green.

ghee   Clarified butter used extensively in Indian cuisine. After the milk solids and water are removed, only pure butterfat remains.

ginger   A flavorful root available fresh or dried and ground that adds a pungent, sweet, and spicy quality to a dish.

goiter   The unnatural enlargement of the thyroid gland that occurs when the thyroid is producing either too much hormone or too little, or sometimes even when it's producing the correct amount (called euthyroidism).

goitrogen   A substance that suppresses the function of the thyroid gland by interfering with iodine uptake, which as a result, can cause an enlargement of the thyroid (a goiter).

Greek yogurt   A strained yogurt that's a good natural source of protein, calcium, and probiotics. Greek yogurt averages 40 percent more protein per ounce than traditional yogurt.

hearts of palm   Firm, elongated, off-white cylinders from the inside of a palm tree stem tip.

herbes de Provence   A seasoning mix of basil, fennel, marjoram, rosemary, sage, and thyme common in the south of France.

Herxheimer reaction   A temporary increase in symptoms when antibiotics or other substances cause a die-off in the offending pathogen that causes the release of toxins and other debris the immune system must reject and remove from the body. Antigens from the debris cause white blood cells to release cellular messengers that induce inflammation and fever.

hoisin sauce   A sweet Asian condiment similar to ketchup made with soybeans, sesame, chile peppers, and sugar.

homeostasis   The body's natural tendency to seek a proper balance in all its systems to maintain health and proper function.

horseradish   A sharp, spicy root that forms the flavor base in condiments such as cocktail sauce and sharp mustards. Prepared horseradish contains vinegar and oil, among other ingredients. Use pure horseradish much more sparingly than the prepared version, or try cutting it with sour cream.

hummus   A thick, Middle Eastern spread made of puréed chickpeas, lemon juice, olive oil, garlic, and often tahini.

inflammation   A condition recognized by the presence of heat, pain, reddened tissue, and swelling.

infusion   A liquid in which flavorful ingredients such as herbs have been soaked or steeped to extract their flavor into the liquid.

Italian seasoning   A blend of dried herbs, including basil, oregano, rosemary, and thyme.

jicama   A juicy, crunchy, sweet, large, round Central American vegetable. If you can't find jicama, try substituting sliced water chestnuts.

julienne   A French word meaning "to slice into very thin pieces."

kalamata olive   Traditionally from Greece, a medium-small, long black olive with a rich, smoky flavor.

keratin   A durable protein polymer found only in epithelial cells. It provides the structural strength to the skin, hair, and nails.

ketoacidosis (diabetic acidocis)   A dangerous condition that may occur in people with diabetes when the body cannot use sugar (glucose) as a fuel source because there's little or no insulin available and fat is used for fuel instead.

kosher salt   A coarse-grained salt made without any additives or iodine.

lentil   A tiny lens-shape pulse used in European, Middle Eastern, and Indian cuisines.

lipoprotein   A particle that transports lipids (fats) around the body in the blood to where they're needed.

litmus paper   pH test paper that's been treated with a natural substance obtained from lichens (mainly *Roccella tinctoria*) so it turns red in response to acidic solutions and blue when exposed to alkaline solutions. In the absence of litmus paper, the raw red cabbage juice can be used to gauge pH. It changes color in response to pH: red = pH 2 (highly acidic), blue = pH 7 (neutral), and greenish-yellow = pH 12 (highly alkaline).

malnutrition   The condition that results from adhering to an unbalanced diet, in which certain nutrients are missing, in excess, or in the wrong proportions.

mandoline   A food-preparation tool used to uniformly slice firm vegetables. With suitable attachments, it can make julienne, crinkle, and waffle cuts as well.

manuka honey   A honey produced in New Zealand by honeybees feeding on the manuka or tea tree that possess amazing antibacterial healing properties.

marjoram   A sweet herb, cousin of and similar to oregano popular in Greek, Spanish, and Italian dishes.

medium-chain triglyceride (MCT)   A 6- to 12-carbon medium-chain fatty acid ester of glycerol (MCFA). MCTs passively move from the GI tract to the portal vein system without the need for modification like long-chain fatty acids (more than 12 carbons) or very-long-chain fatty acids (more than 22 carbons).

meld   To allow flavors to blend and spread over time. Melding is often why recipes call for overnight refrigeration and is also why some dishes taste better as leftovers.

mesclun   Mixed salad greens, usually containing lettuce and other assorted greens such as arugula, cress, and endive.

metabolic syndrome   The name for a cluster of risk factors that increases the chance for coronary artery disease, stroke, and type 2 diabetes.

millet   A tiny, round, yellow-colored nutty-flavored grain often used as a replacement for couscous.

mirin   A type of Japanese rice wine, similar to sake, but with a lower alcohol content.

miso   A fermented, flavorful soybean paste, key in many Japanese dishes.

miso broth   A broth made from miso paste, a thick, salty, tangy base composed of fermented soybeans, barley, rice, or other grains commonly used in Japanese-style soups.

morbidly obese   A condition in which people weigh two or more times their ideal weight and have a BMI of 40 to 49.9. Associated with many serious and life-threatening disorders.

mortar and pestle   A mortar is a sturdy bowl, typically made of ceramic or stone. A pestle is a dense, club-shape tool made of the same material used for crushing, mixing, and grinding hard spices, herbs, or medicines in the mortar.

mouthfeel   The overall sensation in the mouth resulting from a combination of a food's temperature, taste, smell, and texture.

nori   An edible seaweed of the red alga genus *Porphyra*; also known as *laver* in some English-speaking countries. Nori is used extensively in Japanese cuisine, most notably when rolling sushi.

nutmeg   A sweet, fragrant, musky spice used primarily in baking.

obese   A condition in which a person has a BMI of 30 or greater. Obesity results from an abnormal accumulation of body fat and is associated with increased risk of illness, disability, and death.

olive oil   A fragrant liquid produced by crushing or pressing olives. Extra-virgin olive oil—the most flavorful and highest quality—is produced from the first pressing of a batch of olives; oil is also produced from later pressings.

oregano   A fragrant, slightly astringent herb used in Greek, Spanish, and Italian dishes.

orzo   A rice-shape pasta used in Greek cooking.

ossification   The hardening of soft tissue into bonelike material through the process of layering calcium and other mineral deposits.

oxidation   The browning of fruit flesh that happens over time and with exposure to air. Minimize oxidation by rubbing the cut surfaces with lemon juice.

paella   A Spanish dish of rice, shellfish, onion, meats, rich broth, and herbs.

paprika   A rich, red, warm, earthy spice that lends a rich red color to many dishes.

parboil   To partially cook in boiling water or broth.

parsley   A fresh-tasting green, leafy herb, often used as a garnish.

pathogen   Usually a microscopic organism (a germ) such as a virus or bacterium that can cause disease. Fungi and yeast can also become pathogenic.

pathological leukocytosis   An abnormal condition, including elevated white blood cell counts, generally associated with infection, intoxication, poisoning, and eating cooked or abnormally altered foods.

pesto   A thick spread or sauce made with fresh basil leaves, garlic, olive oil, pine nuts, and Parmesan cheese.

pH   The potential of hydrogen. pH refers to the concentration of hydrogen in a solution. A pH of 4 is 10 times more acidic than a pH of 5, and a pH of 5 is 10 times more acidic than a pH of 6, etc. The pH of pure water is normally 7.

phenol   A chemical compound found in plants that contains antioxidants that help protect the body against free radical damage and chronic illnesses.

pilaf　A rice dish in which the rice is browned in butter or oil and then cooked in a flavorful liquid such as a broth, often with the addition of meats or vegetables.

pine nut　A nut that's rich (high in fat), flavorful, and a bit pine-y. Pine nuts are a traditional ingredient in pesto and add a hearty crunch to many other recipes.

pita bread　A flat, hollow wheat bread often used for sandwiches or sliced pizza style. It's terrific soft with dips or baked or broiled as a vehicle for other ingredients.

poach　To cook a food in simmering liquid such as water, wine, or broth.

polenta　A mush made from cornmeal that can be eaten hot with butter or cooked until firm and cut into squares.

polyphenol　An antioxidant found in certain foods that's believed to also affect cell-to-cell signaling, receptor sensitivity, inflammatory enzyme activity, and gene regulation.

porcini mushroom　A rich and flavorful mushroom used in rice and Italian-style dishes.

portobello mushroom　A mature and larger form of the smaller crimini mushroom. Brown, chewy, and flavorful, portobellos are often served as whole caps, grilled, or as thin sautéed slices. *See also* crimini mushrooms.

prosciutto　A dry, salt-cured ham that originated in Italy.

purée　To reduce a food to a thick, creamy texture, typically using a blender or food processor.

queso fresco　"Fresh cheese" in Spanish, queso fresco is an unaged white Mexican cheese made from raw cow's milk, or a mixture of cow's and goat's milk. It has mild, fresh taste similar in some ways to mozzarella.

quinoa　A nutty-flavored seed that's extremely high in protein and calcium.

rapadura   Dehydrated cane sugar juice. Rapadura is a rich source of minerals—especially silica—and is a good substitute for sugar in cookies and cakes.

reduce   To boil or simmer a broth or sauce to remove some of the water content, resulting in more concentrated flavor and color.

rice vinegar   Vinegar produced from fermented rice or rice wine, popular in Asian-style dishes.

risotto   A popular Italian rice dish made by browning arborio rice in butter or oil and then slowly adding liquid to cook the rice, resulting in a creamy texture.

roast   To cook something uncovered in an oven, usually without additional liquid.

rosemary   A pungent, sweet herb used with chicken, pork, fish, and especially lamb. A little goes a long way.

roux   A mixture of butter or another fat and flour, used to thicken sauces and soups.

saffron   An expensive spice made from the stamens of crocus flowers that lends a dramatic yellow color and distinctive flavor to a dish. Use only tiny amounts.

sage   An herb with a musty yet fruity, lemon-rind scent and "sunny" flavor.

sauté   To pan-cook over lower heat than what's used for frying.

savory   A popular herb with a fresh, woody taste. Can also describe the flavor of food.

scald   To heat milk just until it's about to boil and then remove it from heat. Scalding milk helps prevent it from souring.

scant   An ingredient measurement directive not to add any extra, perhaps even leaving the measurement a tad short.

sear   To quickly brown the exterior of a food, especially meat, over high heat.

sesame oil An oil made from pressing sesame seeds. It's tasteless if clear and aromatic and flavorful if brown.

shallot A member of the onion family that grows in a bulb somewhat like garlic but has a milder onion flavor. When a recipe calls for shallot, use the entire bulb.

shiitake mushroom A large, dark brown mushroom with a hearty, meaty flavor. It can be used fresh or dried, grilled, as a component in other recipes, and as a flavoring source for broth.

shiro miso paste A light yellow miso paste commonly known as white miso in the West or summer miso in Japan. It's less salty and undergoes a shorter fermentation period than other misos.

short-grain rice A starchy rice popular in Asian-style dishes because it readily clumps, making it perfect for eating with chopsticks.

simmer To boil a liquid gently so it barely bubbles.

spelt An ancient type of wheat valued for its nutty flavor, high protein, and nutrition content. Spelt contains gluten.

spiralizer A simple, lathelike cutting tool that can fashion spaghetti or flat noodle shapes from raw zucchini, carrots, and other vegetables.

steam To suspend a food over boiling water and allow the heat of the steam (water vapor) to cook the food.

steep To let sit in hot water, as in steeping tea in hot water for 10 minutes.

stew To slowly cook pieces of food submerged in a liquid. Also, a dish prepared by this method.

sticky rice *See* short-grain rice.

stir-fry To cook small pieces of food in a wok or skillet over high heat, moving and turning the food quickly to cook all sides.

stock   A flavorful broth made by cooking meats and/or vegetables with seasonings until the liquid absorbs these flavors. The liquid is strained, and the solids are discarded. Stock can be eaten alone or used as a base for soups, stews, etc.

strata   A savory bread pudding made with eggs and cheese.

tabbouleh   A traditional Arabian salad made of bulgur wheat, chopped tomatoes, parsley, mint, onion, and garlic and marinated in a dressing of olive oil, lemon juice, and salt. Western variations are sometimes made with couscous or quinoa instead of cracked wheat.

tahini   A paste made from sesame seeds, used to flavor many Middle Eastern recipes.

tamari   A naturally fermented premium soy sauce made with extremely little wheat or no wheat at all.

tamarind   A sweet, pungent, flavorful fruit used in Indian-style sauces and curries.

tapenade   A thick, chunky spread made from savory ingredients such as olives, lemon juice, and anchovies.

tarragon   A sweet, rich-smelling herb perfect with seafood, vegetables (especially asparagus), chicken, and pork.

tempeh   An Indonesian food made by culturing and fermenting soybeans into a cake, sometimes mixed with grains or vegetables. It's high in protein and fiber.

teriyaki   A Japanese-style sauce composed of soy sauce, rice wine, ginger, and sugar that works well with seafood as well as most meats.

thyme   A minty, zesty herb.

tofu   A cheeselike substance made from soybeans and soy milk.

turmeric   A spicy, pungent yellow root used in many dishes, especially Indian cuisine, for color and flavor. Turmeric is the source of the yellow color in many prepared mustards.

tzatziki   A Greek dip traditionally made with Greek yogurt, cucumbers, garlic, and mint.

umami A savory flavor, one of the five balancing flavors of Japanese cuisine. The other four are sweet, sour, salty, and bitter.

umeboshi paste A seasoning paste made of pickled Japanese umeboshi (or ume) fruit, a type of plum. The paste is salty, with a sour flavor due to its high citric acid content.

velouté One of the five "mother sauces" in classical French cuisine. It serves as a versatile base for many soups and other sauces.

vichyssoise A classic puréed French soup made of leeks, potatoes, cream, and chicken stock, usually served cold. When served warm, it's known as *potage parmentier*; if it's made without dairy, it's called *potage bonne femme*.

vinegar An acidic liquid widely used as a dressing and seasoning, often made from fermented grapes, apples, or rice. *See also* balsamic vinegar; cider vinegar; rice vinegar; white vinegar; wine vinegar.

wasabi Japanese horseradish, a fiery, pungent condiment used with many Japanese-style dishes. It's most often sold as a powder to which you add water to create a paste.

water chestnut A white, crunchy, and juicy tuber popular in many Asian dishes. It holds its texture whether cool or hot.

whey The liquid milk serum that remains after milk has been curdled and strained—such as in cheese or yogurt making.

whisk To rapidly mix, introducing air to the mixture.

white mushroom A button mushroom. When fresh, white mushrooms have an earthy smell and an appealing soft crunch.

white vinegar The most common type of vinegar, produced from grain.

whole grain A grain derived from the seeds of grasses, including rice, oats, rye, wheat, wild rice, quinoa, barley, buckwheat, bulgur, corn, millet, amaranth, and sorghum.

whole-wheat flour Wheat flour that contains the entire grain.

wild rice Not a rice at all, this grass has a rich, nutty flavor and serves as a nutritious side dish.

wine vinegar   Vinegar produced from red or white wine.

yeast   Tiny fungi that, when mixed with water, sugar, flour, and heat, release carbon dioxide bubbles, which, in turn, cause the bread to rise.

zest   Small slivers of peel, usually from a citrus fruit such as a lemon, lime, or orange.

In this appendix, I share information on where to find various foods items and other products that will make your pH balance diet a more enjoyable experience. I also provide further reading material so you can continue to learn about pH balance nutrition.

Alkalizing Food and Products Sources

Amazing Grass Organic Green SuperFoods
amazinggrass.com
Sells powdered alkalizing nutritional supplements made of certified organic herbs, fruits, and vegetables.

Bob's Red Mill
bobsredmill.com
Sells a wide variety of whole grains and whole-grain flours.

CHEFS
chefscatalog.com
Sells an excellent selection of high-quality food preparation and kitchen equipment, including professional-grade knives, steamers, and juicers.

Eden Foods
edenfoods.com
Sells certified organic foods and canned goods, including whole grains, beans, sea vegetables, cereals, vegetable oils, seed and nut butters, teas, miso, shoyu, umeboshi plums, kuzu root starch, rice vinegar, rice bran pickles, and mirin.

I Shop Indian
ishopindian.com
Sells dahl (dried lentils), grains, spices, oils, and all things Indian.

The Kushi Store
kushistore.com
Sells natural macrobiotic foods, including sea vegetables, whole grains, cereals, beans, seeds, and legumes.

Lundberg Family Farms
lundberg.com
Sells high-quality, certified organic brown rice and brown rice syrup.

Maine Coast Sea Vegetables
seaveg.com
Sells certified organic, sustainably harvested sea vegetables and sea vegetable products of all kinds.

Melissa's Produce
melissas.com
Sells fresh young coconut, mature coconut, and excellent produce of every kind.

Mt. Capra Wholefood Nutritionals
mtcapra.com
Sells high-potassium dehydrated goat milk whey.

NOW Foods
nowfoods.com
Sells Green Phyto-Foods made from green plants, cereal grasses, and algae in tablet and powder form.

pH Sciences
phsciences.com
Sells pH Balance, an alkalizing blend of minerals (calcium, magnesium, and potassium) in tablet form.

Thai Supermarket Online
importfood.com
Sells hard-to-find noodles, spices, oils, sauces, and all things Thai.

Tropical Traditions

tropicaltraditions.com

Sells organic virgin and expeller-pressed coconut oil, coconut cream concentrate, flaked coconut, red palm oil, coconut vinegar, coconut flour, organic free-range bison and poultry, raw dairy, and raw Canadian honey.

WheatgrassKits.com

wheatgrasskits.com

Sells organic, live, whole-food products, including kits for growing wheatgrass, barleygrass, sunflower greens, sprouts, and herbs, as well as a good selection of juicers.

Young Coconuts

youngcoconuts.com

Sells coconut openers, coconut shredders, coconut de-meaters, coconut scrapers, and the Coconut Noodle Maker.

Online Resources

Blanco Botanicals

blancobotanicals.com

My website. Includes holistic nutrition consulting, education, medicinal herb information, natural health articles, and a health and wellness blog.

Melissa's Produce

tinyurl.com/bm72kc7

Provides recipes using fresh coconut and other fresh produce.

Nutrition and Physical Degeneration

gutenberg.net.au/ebooks02/0200251h.html

The research of Dr. Weston A. Price.

The Oiling of America

tinyurl.com/6taedow

Scholarly articles by Mary G. Enig, PhD, and Sally Fallon.

Price-Pottenger Nutrition Foundation

ppnf.org

Orthomolecular resources and education related to restoring physical and mental health through nutrition and other natural means.

The Weston A. Price Foundation
westonaprice.org
Scholarly health and nutrition articles.

Further Reading

Bowden, Jonny, PhC, CNS. *The 150 Healthiest Foods on Earth.* Gloucester, MA: Fair Winds Press, 2007.

Brown, Susan E., and Larry Trivieri Jr., *The Acid Alkaline Food Guide.* Garden City Park, NY: Square One Publishers, 2006.

Calbom, Cherie, MS. *The Ultimate Smoothie Book: 130 Delicious Recipes for Blender Drinks, Frozen Desserts, Shakes, and More!* New York, NY: Grand Central Life and Style, 2001.

Cook, Michelle Schoffro, DNM, DAc, CNC. *The Ultimate pH Solution.* New York, NY: HarperCollins, 2008.

Daniel, Kaayla T., PhD, CCN. *The Whole Soy Story.* Washington, DC: New Trends Publishing, 2005.

Fallon, Sally, and Mary G. Enig, PhD. *Nourishing Traditions.* Washington, DC: New Trends Publishing, 2001.

Gerson, Charlotte, and Morton Walker. *The Gerson Therapy.* New York, NY: Kensington Publishing, 2001.

Mateljan, George. *The World's Healthiest Foods.* Seattle, WA: George Mateljan Foundation, 2007.

Price, Weston A., DDS. *Nutrition and Physical Degeneration.* La Mesa, CA: Keats, 1939.

Ross, Bonnie. *The Amazing Acid Alkaline Cookbook.* Garden City Park, NY: Square One Publishers, 2011.

Shilhavey, Brian, and Marianita Shilhavey. *Virgin Coconut Oil.* West Bend, WI: Tropical Traditions, 2004.

Vasey, Christopher, NC. *The Acid Alkaline Diet for Optimum Health.* Rochester, VT: Healing Arts Press, 2006.

Whang, Sang. *Reverse Aging.* Miami, FL: JSP Publishing, 1990.

Food Tables

I included this appendix as a resource to help you determine which foods are relatively more alkalizing or acidifying in your diet. As you work to maintain a healthy alkaline balance, be sure to stay hydrated by drinking plenty of water.

Monitor your internal pH as described in Chapter 4, and use that reading as a guide in selecting what foods you combine for any given meal. The more acidic your pH reading, the more alkaline-producing foods you should eat. If your readings are only slightly acidic or slightly alkaline (pH = 6.5 to 7.5), 60 to 65 percent of your plate (visually, about two-thirds, or from noon to 8 on a clock face) should hold alkaline-producing foods. If your readings are moderately (pH = 6.0 to 6.4) to extremely acidic (pH = 5.0 or less), at least 80 percent of your plate should hold alkaline-producing foods (visually, $\frac{4}{5}$ or from noon to 10 on a clock face).

While on a pH balance diet, most of your food selections should come from the alkaline columns. But that doesn't mean you can never eat more acidic foods. Try to keep the acid-forming foods down to approximately 20 percent of your total intake in any given meal or snack, and be sure to include plenty of raw vegetables and juices.

Alkalizing and Acidifying Foods

Food or Drink	Highly Acid Forming	Moderately Acid Forming	Mildly Acid Forming	Mildly Alkaline Forming	Moderately Alkaline Forming	Highly Alkaline Forming
Açai berries			X			
Agave nectar			X			
Alcohol sugar-based sweeteners (malatol, xylatol, etc.)		X				
Alfalfa, juiced grass or sprouts					X	X
Algae, blue-green, freeze-dried			X			
Almond butter, raw				X		
Almond milk, sweetened			X	X		
Almond milk, unsweetened				X		
Almonds				X		
Amaranth, flour			X			
Amaranth, grain			X			
Apple butter					X	
Apple cider					X	
Apple cider vinegar					X	
Apple juice, sweetened			X			

Food or Drink	Highly Acid Forming	Moderately Acid Forming	Mildly Acid Forming	Mildly Alkaline Forming	Moderately Alkaline Forming	Highly Alkaline Forming
Apple juice, unsweetened				X	X	
Apples			X			
Apricots, dried			X			
Apricots, fresh			X			
Artichokes				X		
Artificial sweeteners (aspartame, saccharine, etc.)	X					
Asparagus				X		
Avocados					X	
Baking soda					X	
Bananas, green				X		
Bananas, ripe		X				
Barley			X			
Barley grass, juiced						X
Barley malt sweetener			X			
Barley malt syrup			X			
Basil				X		
Bee pollen				X		
Beef	X					

continues

Alkalizing and Acidifying Foods (continued)

Food or Drink	Highly Acid Forming	Moderately Acid Forming	Mildly Acid Forming	Mildly Alkaline Forming	Moderately Alkaline Forming	Highly Alkaline Forming
Beer	X					
Beets, fresh red					X	
Bell peppers				X		
Blackberries			X			
Blueberries			X			
Bok choy				X		
Borage oil				X		
Brazil nuts			X			
Bread, rye			X			
Bread (most)	X	X				
Breakfast cereals, cold, processed		X				
Brown rice syrup			X			
Brussels sprouts				X		
Buffalo		X				
Bulgur wheat			X			
Burdock root						X
Butter			X			
Cabbage, green				X		
Cabbage, red				X		
Cabbage, savoy				X		
Cabbage, white				X		

Food or Drink	Highly Acid Forming	Moderately Acid Forming	Mildly Acid Forming	Mildly Alkaline Forming	Moderately Alkaline Forming	Highly Alkaline Forming
Cake, cookies, etc. (store-bought)	X					
Cantaloupe			X			
Caraway seeds				X		
Carbonated drinks (most)	X					
Carrots				X		
Cashews			X			
Cauliflower				X		
Cayenne					X	
Celery					X	
Cheese, American	X					
Cheese, most, but especially firm, aged cheeses	X					
Cherimoya			X			
Cherries, sour				X		
Cherries, sweet			X			
Chestnuts				X		
Chicken		X				
Chives						X
Chocolate candies		X				
Cilantro					X	

continues

Alkalizing and Acidifying Foods   (continued)

Food or Drink	Highly Acid Forming	Moderately Acid Forming	Mildly Acid Forming	Mildly Alkaline Forming	Moderately Alkaline Forming	Highly Alkaline Forming
Clementines			X			
Coconut, fresh				X		
Coconut oil, virgin				X		
Cod liver oil			X			
Coffee	X					
Coffee substitutes, grain based			X			
Comfrey				X		
Couscous			X			
Cranberries			X			
Cream, dairy			X			
Cucumbers						X
Cumin seeds				X		
Currants			X			
Dandelion, greens and root						X
Dates			X			
Duck		X				
Egg whites		X				
Eggplant (aubergine)				X		
Eggs, whole		X				

Food or Drink	Highly Acid Forming	Moderately Acid Forming	Mildly Acid Forming	Mildly Alkaline Forming	Moderately Alkaline Forming	Highly Alkaline Forming
Endive						
Evening primrose oil				X	X	
Farina	X					
Fennel seeds				X		
Figs, dried				X		
Figs, raw				X		
Fish, fresh water		X				
Fish, salt water		X				
Flaxseed oil				X		
Flaxseeds			X			
Frozen vegetables, processed (most)		X				
Fructose		X				
Fruit juice, raw			X			
Fruit juice, sweetened	X					
Garlic					X	
Ginger					X	
Ginseng				X		
Goji berries			X			
Gooseberries			X			
Grapefruit			X			

continues

Alkalizing and Acidifying Foods   (continued)

Food or Drink	Highly Acid Forming	Moderately Acid Forming	Mildly Acid Forming	Mildly Alkaline Forming	Moderately Alkaline Forming	Highly Alkaline Forming
Grapes			X			
Green beans					X	
Grits, corn		X				
Halva		X				
Hazelnuts (filberts)			X			
Honey			X			
Horseradish			X	X		
Hummus			X			
Jicama						X
Kale						X
Kamut				X		
Kamut grass, juiced						X
Ketchup		X				
Kohlrabi				X		
Lactose (milk sugar)			X			
Lambs' lettuce				X		
Leeks				X		
Lemons				X		
Lentils				X		
Lettuce				X		

Food or Drink	Highly Acid Forming	Moderately Acid Forming	Mildly Acid Forming	Mildly Alkaline Forming	Moderately Alkaline Forming	Highly Alkaline Forming
Lima beans					X	
Limes				X		
Liquor	X					
Liver			X			
Macadamia nuts			X			
Mandarine oranges		X				
Mangoes			X			
Maple syrup			X			
Margarine			X			
Milk, homogenized			X			
Milk, pasteurized		X				
Milk, raw			X			
Miso					X	X
Molasses		X				
Mushrooms			X	X		
Mustard greens				X		
Navy beans					X	
Nectarines			X			

continues

Alkalizing and Acidifying Foods   (continued)

Food or Drink	Highly Acid Forming	Moderately Acid Forming	Mildly Acid Forming	Mildly Alkaline Forming	Moderately Alkaline Forming	Highly Alkaline Forming
Oatmeal, unsweetened, old-fashioned (prepared)				X		
Oats, whole groats, steel-cut, and Scottish			X			
Olive oil, extra-virgin (raw) and other grades (if raw or in light cooking)				X		
Onions				X		
Oranges			X			
Oregano					X	
Organ meats			X			
Oysters			X			
Paneer		X				
Papayas, ripe			X			
Parsnips				X		
Peaches			X			
Pears			X			
Peanut butter, raw organic		X				

Food or Drink	Highly Acid Forming	Moderately Acid Forming	Mildly Acid Forming	Mildly Alkaline Forming	Moderately Alkaline Forming	Highly Alkaline Forming
Peanuts		X				
Peas				X		
Peppers, bell and chile				X		
Pine nuts				X		
Pineapple		X				
Pistachios		X				
Plums			X			
Pomegranates		X				
Popping corn			X			
Pork	X					
Potatoes				X		
Pumpkin				X		
Pumpkin seeds			X			
Quark cheese		X				
Radishes, diakon						X
Radishes, red					X	
Radishes, summer black						X
Radishes, white spring				X		
Raspberries		X				
Rhubarb				X		

continues

Alkalizing and Acidifying Foods   (continued)

Food or Drink	Highly Acid Forming	Moderately Acid Forming	Mildly Acid Forming	Mildly Alkaline Forming	Moderately Alkaline Forming	Highly Alkaline Forming
Rice, basmati		X				
Rice, brown				X		
Rice milk			X			
Rose hips		X				
Royal jelly			X			
Rutabagas				X		
Sardines, canned	X					
Sauerkraut (vinegar-processed, pasteurized)		X				
Sea vegetables (kelp, hiziki, arame, kombu, nori, etc.)				X		
Sesame oil				X		
Sesame seeds				X		
Soft drinks	X					
Sorrel					X	
Spelt				X		
Spinach				X	X	
Sprouts (grasses, beans, seeds)						X
Strawberries			X			
Sugar, beet		X				

Food or Drink	Highly Acid Forming	Moderately Acid Forming	Mildly Acid Forming	Mildly Alkaline Forming	Moderately Alkaline Forming	Highly Alkaline Forming
Sugar, dried cane juice			X			
Sugar, white, brown, turbinado		X				
Sunflower oil			X			
Sunflower seeds			X			
Sweet potatoes			X			
Tangerines			X			
Tea, black	X					
Tea, herbal or green				X		
Tempeh			X			
Thyme				X		
Tofu				X	X	
Tomatoes, cooked					X	
Tomatoes, raw				X		
Tuna, canned	X					
Turnips				X		
Veal	X					
Vegetables, canned		X				
Vegetables, fresh cooked (most)			X			

continues

Alkalizing and Acidifying Foods (continued)

Food or Drink	Highly Acid Forming	Moderately Acid Forming	Mildly Acid Forming	Mildly Alkaline Forming	Moderately Alkaline Forming	Highly Alkaline Forming
Vegetables, pickled (vinegar-processed, pasteurized)	X					
Vinegar, apple cider			X			
Walnuts			X			
Water, mineral				X		
Water, sparkling		X				
Water, spring			X			
Watercress				X		
Watermelon			X			
Wheat		X				
Wheat kernel		X				
Wheatgrass, juiced						X
Whey protein powder			X			
Wine		X				
Yams				X		
Yeast			X			
Yogurt, plain			X			
Yogurt, sweetened		X				
Zucchini				X		

Relative Acid/Alkaline Forming Foods by Type

Food by Type	Very Acid Forming	Moderately Acid Forming	Mildly Acid Forming	Mildly Alkaline Forming	Moderately Alkaline Forming	Very Alkaline Forming
Beverages	Alcohol (wine, beer, spirits), coffee, fruit juice (sweetened/ processed), black tea, soft drinks, sports/energy drinks	Fruit juices (raw, unprocessed)		Distilled water		Mineral water, water alkalized with lemon/lime juice, vegetable juices (fresh, raw)
Condiments	Carob, cocoa, fruit jams/jellies/ preserves, malts, prepared mustard, rice syrup, soy sauce, vinegars (most)	Ketchup, mayonnaise				
Dairy products and substitutes	Casein, cheeses, ice cream, whey, yogurt		Cow's milk, cream, rice milk	Almond milk, coconut milk, goat's milk		Human breast milk

continues

Relative Acid/Alkaline Forming Foods by Type   (continued)

Food by Type	Very Acid Forming	Moderately Acid Forming	Mildly Acid Forming	Mildly Alkaline Forming	Moderately Alkaline Forming	Very Alkaline Forming
Fats and oils	Margarine	Canola oil, corn oil	Butter, grapeseed oil, soybean oil, sunflower oil, walnut oil	Almond oil, avocado oil, borage oil, coconut oil, cod liver oil, evening primrose oil, flaxseed oil, olive oil		
Fish, meat and poultry	Beef, eggs, fish (farmed), pork, shellfish, veal	Fish (wild-caught, saltwater)	Fish (wild-caught, freshwater)			
Fruit	Processed, dried, pickled, or canned fruit	Apples, apricots, bananas, berries, currants, figs, grapes (and raisins), guava, honeydew melon, mangoes, oranges, papayas (ripe), peaches, pears, persimmon, pineapple, satsumas, sweet cherries, tangerines, watermelon	Cantaloupe, dates, nectarines, plums	Coconut, grapefruit, lemons, limes, sour cherries, tomatoes	Avocados	

Food by Type	Very Acid Forming	Moderately Acid Forming	Mildly Acid Forming	Mildly Alkaline Forming	Moderately Alkaline Forming	Very Alkaline Forming
Grains	Barley, corn, oat bran	Breads (white, whole-grain, rye), oats, rice (brown, wild)	Amaranth, kasha, millet	Buckwheat, quinoa, spelt		
Herbs and spices		Nutmeg, table salt, vanilla extract			Cayenne, dried and fresh herbs (parsley, sage, rosemary, thyme, etc.)	Himalayan salt, sea salt
Legumes	Peanuts		Black beans, chickpeas (garbanzo beans), kidney beans	Lentils, tofu	Lima beans, navy beans	
Seeds and nuts	Cashews, pistachios	Walnuts	Brazil nuts, hazelnuts (filberts), pecans, flaxseeds, sunflower seeds	Almonds (raw), caraway seeds, cumin seeds, fennel seeds, sesame seeds		Pumpkin seeds (pepitas)

continues

Relative Acid/Alkaline Forming Foods by Type   (continued)

Food by Type	Very Acid Forming	Moderately Acid Forming	Mildly Acid Forming	Mildly Alkaline Forming	Moderately Alkaline Forming	Very Alkaline Forming
Sweeteners	Agave nectar, artificial sweeteners, beet sugar, corn syrup, honey, molasses, rice syrup, white sugar			Stevia		
Vegetables	Potatoes (russet, red, white)			Artichokes, asparagus, Brussels sprouts, carrots, cauliflower, chives, horseradish, kohlrabi, leeks, rhubarb, rutabagas, sweet peas, sweet potatoes, turnips, turnip greens, watercress, yams, zucchini	Arugula, beets, broccoli, cabbage, collard greens, endive, garlic, ginger, green beans, hot peppers, mustard greens, okra, onions, radishes, salad greens, sorrel, spinach, sweet peppers	Cucumbers, dandelion greens, kale, sea vegetables (dulse, wakame, kombu, arame, nori, hijiki, kelp, agar agar, bladderwrack), bean sprouts (raw), seed sprouts (raw)

Your Personalized pH Balance Diet Profile

For this exercise, you need your journal and either the photos or food packaging you've collected over the course of a week. Read and thoughtfully consider each of the following points. Answer the questions honestly, and your unique profile will emerge.

Look at your journal, and estimate what percentage of fresh food you usually eat.   Ideally, 75 to 80 percent of the food you eat should be fresh foods—either cooked or raw. If your percentage of fresh foods is relatively low, increase the number of meals you eat that contain fresh ingredients. What is your goal? Write it down.

On average, how many servings of vegetables do you eat per day?   Each day, strive to eat five servings of vegetables—at a *minimum*. Vegetables are key in balancing your pH and reducing your risk for many diseases. Do you eat more than that? Bravo! Determine what, if any, changes you need to make, and write them down.

Generally speaking, is your diet varied? Or do you eat the same things every day?   If you eat the same things again and again—even if the food is healthy—you are missing nutrients in your diet. Repeatedly consuming the same foods also raises your risk of developing food allergies. Strive to limit your favorite foods to a four-day rotation to promote better nutrition and reduce the risk of allergies.

How much fast food have do you eat?   Fast food and many restaurant meals are full of trans fats, excess salt, sugar, and artificial ingredients—all of which wreak havoc with your pH. Does your fast-food consumption need adjustment? Write down what you plan to do.

How much sugar and salt do you eat?   Read the nutrition
information labels you collected for an eye-opening experience.
Then consider the sugar you add to your coffee and tea and the
salt you sprinkle over your dinner plate. Processed foods are full of
added sugar, salt, and dangerous artificial sweeteners. Reducing these
foods goes a long way toward balancing your pH, and replacing salt
and sugar with herbs, spices, and citrus juices enhances your food's
flavor and increases nutrition at the same time. Look at your journal,
decide what improvements you can make, and write them down.

How many bread and wheat products do you consume?   Wheat
products aggravate blood sugar stability and contain gluten, which
may lead to serious digestive problems. Wheat also contains opioids
that contribute to developing allergic addictions that negatively affect
brain function. Consider reducing your wheat consumption and
substituting other whole grains, such as millet, barley, brown rice,
and amaranth, in its place. Write down a plan for how you can avoid
the overconsumption of wheat in the future.

What is your percentage of good fats to bad fats?   You should
be emphasizing omega-3 fatty acids, found in cold-water fatty fish
(salmon, sardines, and so on.); organic butter; naturally saturated
MCT fats like virgin coconut oil; and fats that naturally occur in
olives, seeds, and nuts. Hydrogenated trans fats and polyunsaturated
oils cause inflammation and free radical formation that's unhealthy
and causes acidification in the body. Consider what changes you can
make to increase good fats while decreasing bad fats in your diet, and
write them down.

Are you addicted to caffeine?   Generally speaking, there's
nothing wrong with having a cup of coffee, but many people take it
to extremes. Caffeine wreaks havoc with your nerves and exhausts
your adrenal glands, leaving you feeling exhausted and carrying extra
weight around your middle. Decaffeinated coffees aren't the answer
because they contain chemical solvents that, among other things,
mess with your pH. Consider substituting plenty of pure water and
health-promoting herbal teas instead. Write down how you plan to
manage caffeine.

Are you a snacker?   Snacking is good for you—*if* you choose the right snacks. Fruits, vegetables, nuts, and seeds provide intense nutrition, excellent amounts of fiber, and the good fats and pure water your body needs. Chips, cookies, candies, cakes, and ice creams, however, contain far too much acid-forming potential to be of use in balancing your pH. Decide which healthful snacks you'd like to add to your diet, and write them down.

Do you drink alcohol?   The occasional glass of wine likely won't cause problems, but excessive consumption of alcohol stimulates the appetite, weakens the liver, and contributes to weight gain and acid pH. Decide how you can manage or eliminate alcohol consumption, and write that down.

Now take a look at yourself in the mirror and write down your goals. Goals are highly personal, specific outcomes you desire. Examples might be: "I want to feel more relaxed and less frazzled all the time," "I want to be slim," or "I want bright, clear eyes and radiant skin." Don't limit yourself to only what you think is possible—list all your goals, and know that they're obtainable. The pH balance diet profile you just outlined can help. You can get there if you try!

Assessing Your Journey

After the end of your 28-day pH balance journey, gather your journal and notes, and come back to this section to assess how well you've done. I bet you'll be pleasantly surprised.

Consider the following questions, and record your answers, feelings, and impressions:

What is the percentage of fresh food in your diet now?

How much has your consumption of raw fruits and vegetables increased?

Are you drinking more water and less caffeinated, sugary, or alcoholic beverages?

Have you made an improvement in the snacks you eat?

Do you eat a greater variety now?

How do you feel now compared to how you felt before?

Have you had a medical checkup? Did your vitals improve?

How have your energy levels, digestion, and quality of sleep changed?

Look at yourself in the mirror. What changes do you see in your body, face, and hair? How do your clothes fit? Do you look and feel sexy?

Has your mood improved? Are you happier, calmer?

Are you finding time for exercise and relaxation?

If you feel good about the results you've achieved, you're on the right track! If you feel you still have a way to go to achieve your goals, hang in there—persistence and minor tweaking when necessary are key.

If, on the other hand, you're a little disappointed in your results, use your profile and your answers to guide you in how you can best add more pH-balancing foods and activities. By continuing to add more positive aspects to your foods and your lifestyle, you can continue to edge out the bad.

Index

T

X-Y-Z

CHECK OUT THESE
BEST-SELLERS

More than 450 titles available at booksellers and online retailers everywhere!

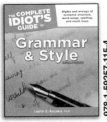
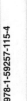
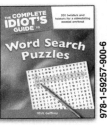
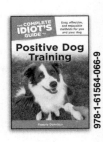
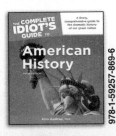
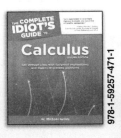
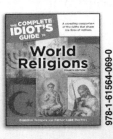
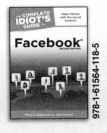
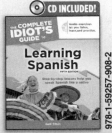
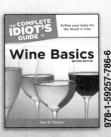
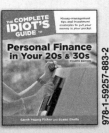
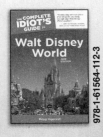
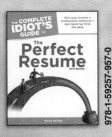
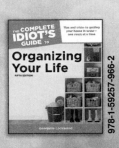
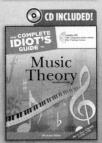